# Using Insulin Pumps
# in Diabetes

# Using Insulin Pumps in Diabetes

*A Guide for Nurses and
Other Health Professionals*

**Jill Rodgers**

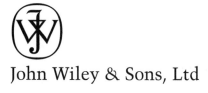

John Wiley & Sons, Ltd

Published by John Wiley & Sons, Ltd, The Atrium, Southern Gate, Chichester,
West Sussex PO19 8SQ, England
Telephone    (+44) 1243 779777

Email (for orders and customer service enquiries): cs-books@wiley.co.uk
Visit our Home Page on www.wiley.com

*Other Wiley Editorial Offices*

John Wiley & Sons Inc., 111 River Street, Hoboken, NJ 07030, USA

Jossey-Bass, 989 Market Street, San Francisco, CA 94103-1741, USA

Wiley-VCH Verlag GmbH, Boschstr. 12, D-69469 Weinheim, Germany

John Wiley & Sons Australia Ltd, 42 McDougall Street, Milton, Queensland 4064, Australia

John Wiley & Sons (Asia) Pte Ltd, 2 Clementi Loop #02-01, Jin Xing Distripark, Singapore 129809

John Wiley & Sons Canada Ltd, 22 Worcester Road, Etobicoke, Ontario, Canada, M9W 1LI

Wiley also publishes its books in a variety of electronic formats. Some content that appears in print may
not be available in electronic books.

*Library of Congress Cataloging-in-Publication Data is available*

Rodgers, Jill.
    Using insulin pumps in diabetes : a guide for nurses and other health professionals / Jill Rodgers.
        p.    ;   cm.
    Includes bibliographical references and index.
    ISBN 978-0-470-05925-8 (pbk. : alk. paper)
  1. Insulin pumps.    2. Diabetes–Treatment.    3. Diabetes–Nursing.    I. Title.
    [DNLM: 1. Insulin Infusion Systems.    2. Diabetes Mellitus–drug therapy.    3. Diabetes Mellitus–nursing.
    4. Insulin–therapeutic use. WK 820 R691u 2008]
    RC661.I63R63 2008
    616.4′620231–dc22                                                                                          2007044833

*British Library Cataloguing in Publication Data*

A catalogue record for this book is available from the British Library

ISBN 9780470059258

Typeset in 10/12.5pt Palatino by Aptara Inc., New Delhi, India
Printed and bound in Great Britain by TJ International Ltd, Padstow, Cornwall
This book is printed on acid-free paper responsibly manufactured from sustainable forestry
in which at least two trees are planted for each one used for paper production.

# Contents

# Foreword

For people living with Type 1 diabetes, the days of fixed insulin doses, twice-daily mixtures and once-a-week blood glucose monitoring should be confined to the dustbin of history. As with many aspects of life, technology continues to advance to help people deal with the nuances of living with a long-term condition.

Over recent years, insulin pump therapy in the United Kingdom has undergone something of a renaissance. Part of the reason for this has involved advances in technology, patient selection and the availability of analogue insulins. Nevertheless, the most important driver for expanding access to this form of therapy has been the enthusiasm and determination of a small group of experienced diabetes specialist nurses. Jill Rodgers has been and continues to be a very prominent member of this group. As in many areas of clinical care, the evidence on which to make decisions about diabetes-related treatment changes needs to be expanded: practical, clinically based experience is vital in order to advise people with diabetes properly.

Throughout the recent expansion of pump therapy, the available literature has been mostly based on US experiences and uses the language of that country, which does not always easily travel across the Atlantic. Although adequate up to a point, there remain significant transatlantic differences in approaches to diabetes education and training. *Using Insulin Pumps in Diabetes: A Guide for Nurses and Other Health Professionals* is a most welcome addition to the literature on insulin pump therapy. Importantly, it is based on many years of experience of dealing with the roller coaster of establishing a pump service and should be compulsory reading for anyone interested in moving into this area. For those already involved, there is always more to learn.

However, it is people with diabetes who will ultimately benefit the most from this book as the access to well-run, innovative and technologically efficient specialist diabetes services should improve exponentially and be available to everyone and anyone with Type 1 diabetes.

*Dr David Kerr*
Consultant Physician and Visiting Professor
Bournemouth Diabetes and Endocrine Centre

# Preface

Continuous subcutaneous insulin infusion, or CSII, therapy is commonly referred to as 'insulin pump therapy' or simply 'pump therapy', and these are the terms that will be used throughout this book.

Insulin pump therapy is now used more widely across the United Kingdom. This is partly due to the accurate and sophisticated technology that modern insulin pumps offer and partly to health professionals becoming more confident in using this type of therapy successfully. Diabetes specialist nurses, dietitians and specialist medical staff play a predominant role in helping people to manage their diabetes using insulin pumps, and this book will provide help to any health professionals working with people with diabetes who are using, or hoping to use, an insulin pump. It provides information that will take the reader step by step through both simple and also more intricate situations that they might come across.

As the author of this book, I am hoping to convey two messages, which might appear to conflict. The first is that insulin pumps can be the key to freedom to those using them: they can find they no longer have to regulate their mealtimes, eat when they are not hungry or live in fear of hypoglycaemic episodes occurring without warning. People can do anything they want to when they use an insulin pump, as there is to some extent a certain amount of simplicity about the whole process – they can increase or decrease their insulin doses to more tightly match their body's insulin needs – so that they can better manage their diabetes in any situation.

The second message is that people can only gain this freedom by learning more about their diabetes: about the general effects of changes to their insulin doses and, through experimentation, about what specific changes work best for them as individuals. So using an insulin pump is not an easy ride; rather, it requires commitment, determination and sheer hard work if an individual is to get the most out of it, and many pump users find the first few weeks or months of using an insulin pump daunting. It also requires willingness on the part of health professionals to develop support systems to help people manage their diabetes using insulin pumps.

My personal view is that an insulin pump should be seen as an essential part of the 'diabetes toolkit'. It is not something that is required or wanted by all, but something that should be used in specific circumstances, with clarity about what is to be gained by using the therapy. Both the health professional and the person with diabetes need to be clear about why a pump might be a suitable option, what the drawbacks are, what commitment is required and also what circumstances might dictate that pump therapy has not worked for that individual.

This book comprehensively covers: the rationale for pump use, how to set up a service to support insulin pump use, how to make decisions about whether a pump is suitable for someone, how to manage insulin doses, food intake and blood glucose levels and how to deal with both everyday situations and those requiring more complex management. Much of its content comes from practical experience: through my own professional experience of working with insulin pumps, through liaison with experienced specialist pump teams across the United Kingdom and also, very importantly, from the comments and feedback of pump users themselves.

In many areas of pump management, there is a paucity of evidence, and also opinions vary between specialist teams regarding how to manage different situations. This book will not dictate exactly what to do in every situation, simply because there are often a number of choices of actions to take. Instead, this book offers a range of options to choose from to manage pump therapy, and as they gain expertise pump users and health professionals will also develop alternative ways of dealing with specific situations, in addition to those discussed in this book.

*Jill Rodgers*

# Acknowledgements

There are a number of people to whom I would like to offer thanks for their help and support in writing this book.

First, my brilliant team of reviewers of diabetes specialist dietitians and nurses, who gave me objective comments on my work as it progressed and answered my queries promptly. They are: Mary Bilous (Middlesbrough), Joan Everett (Bournemouth), Carole Gelder (Leeds), Emma Jenkins (Bournemouth) and Gill Morrison (Liverpool).

Second, people with diabetes who use, or have thought about using, insulin pump therapy. This book is shaped by the people I have come in contact with over the years, but particular thanks go to Mike Barker, Stuart Bootle, Julie Brickley, Kirsty Samuel, Joe Solowiejczyk and Claire Welling for sharing their individual thoughts and experiences with me during the writing of this book.

I would also like to thank all the companies involved in insulin pump therapy for their support and help with information to ensure this book is factually correct. Again, there have been many people, but particular thanks go to Steven Baard (Roche Diagnostics Ltd), John Hughes (Advanced Therapeutics Ltd) and Julia Shaw (Medtronic Ltd).

Finally, I also wanted to acknowledge the huge support I got from people close to me, and in particular two people who have believed in my ability to write this book and have given me encouragement at every stage. First, Mike Carpenter, my partner, whose objective comments and help have been invaluable. Second, Rosie Walker, my business partner, who has also supported me throughout and has helped me find the time I have needed to write this book.

All the people I have named here are but a few of the many who have offered help, support and advice along the way, and whose experiences have helped make this book what it is. Thank you.

# Chapter 1
# An Introduction to Insulin Pump Therapy

This chapter will provide information on what insulin pump therapy is, and how insulin pumps have developed from the early models introduced in the 1970s to the sophisticated models in use today. National guidance on the use of insulin pumps in the United Kingdom will be discussed, as will alternative devices that are either being researched or are in limited use. It is likely that technological advances will result in many new devices being developed over the next decade. More detailed information on all aspects of insulin pump therapy can be found in the relevant sections throughout this book.

## WHAT IS INSULIN PUMP THERAPY?

Insulin pump therapy, also known as 'continuous subcutaneous insulin infusion' (or CSII) therapy, is a method of giving insulin subcutaneously without the need for injections. In brief, a small needle or catheter is introduced and left in place under the skin, and the insulin pump is attached to this via a length of tubing. The needle or catheter needs to be replaced every two to three days for most people. The pump is worn 24 hours a day (although can be removed for short periods) and delivers fast-acting insulin continuously, in very small amounts, known as the 'basal rate'. The amount of insulin being delivered is programmed by the individual pump user according to their needs. Additional insulin doses, known as 'boluses', are given by the pump user – for example when they are eating or if their blood glucose level is too high – by pressing buttons on the pump in sequence.

## THE DEVELOPMENT OF INSULIN PUMP THERAPY

Historically, insulin pump therapy first became an option for treating diabetes in the 1970s. Technology at that time was very limited, so, although they provided a continuous supply of insulin and provided the opportunity to give boluses without additional injections, insulin pumps lacked the sophistication of modern-day pumps, and were only capable of delivering boluses as multiples of the basal rate. Dose adjustment for many pumps could only be achieved through using a screwdriver to turn a screw head. The pumps delivered the insulin boluses slowly, over about 20 minutes. The devices were also significantly larger than today's models and lacked adequate alarm systems to identify when they were malfunctioning or not delivering the programmed insulin, thereby increasing the risk of diabetic ketoacidosis.

In addition, health professionals lacked the knowledge and skills needed to optimise the effect of insulin delivered via a pump, and people using the pumps were not given the training and support that they needed. Pumps were used to treat people with diabetes in whom all other therapies were deemed to have failed, so the pump was viewed as a last resort rather than as a proactive management choice. No assessment of interest or enthusiasm for using a pump was made of people before pump therapy was initiated, and, together with the lack of education, this meant that in general insulin pumps were poorly managed. As one of the most common side effects was diabetic ketoacidosis, insulin pump therapy was viewed as a treatment option that carried with it more disadvantages than advantages. Even though analysis reported that insulin pumps carried no greater risk of mortality than conventional therapy (Teutsch *et al.*, 1984), the myth that pump therapy is less reliable than injection therapy has resulted in many healthcare providers being reluctant to use it in clinical practice (Saudek, 1997), and might have contributed to the slow growth in the use of this therapy in the United Kingdom.

## TODAY'S INSULIN PUMPS

Modern insulin pumps, in line with other electronic devices, have become extremely sophisticated. They deliver insulin in tiny quantities, down to as little as 0.025 units per hour, and can be programmed to deliver insulin much more physiologically than multiple-dose insulin therapy. While from a safety aspect they generally require a series of button-pressing to alter insulin doses or give additional doses, they are much more straightforward to use than their predecessors. Information about the current pumps available and their range of features is available in Chapter Four.

The improvement in technology is one aspect that makes insulin pump therapy a success today, but there are also other factors, in particular the recognition that careful assessment of individuals is required prior to their using a pump, which is discussed further in Chapter Six. The provision of intensive education and ongoing support from a specialist team is also important and helps people to optimise their diabetes management when using a pump. In the Diabetes Control and Complications Trial, carried out in the United States between 1984 and 1993, 42 per cent of those in the intensively treated group were using insulin pump therapy by the end of the trial (Diabetes Control and Complications Trial Research Group, 1993), indicating the potential it has for optimising glycaemic control.

As a result of the problems experienced in the 1970s and early 1980s, insulin pumps have been used with a great deal of caution in the United Kingdom. In addition, in the UK healthcare system, essential treatments are traditionally funded much more readily than those that are viewed to have cheaper alternatives, in this case injection therapy. The number of people in the United Kingdom who currently use insulin pumps to manage their diabetes has risen from under 200 in 1998 (Everett, 2003) to 5000–6000 in 2006 (Diabetes UK, 2006), and this number continues to rise. This means that 2 per cent or more of the UK population who have Type 1 diabetes currently use insulin pumps to manage their diabetes, compared with 15–20 per cent of people in the United States and some parts of Europe.

## National guidance on insulin pump therapy

The National Institute for Health and Clinical Excellence (NICE) produced guidance in 2003 (National Institute for Health and Clinical Excellence, 2003) on the use of insulin pump therapy, outlined in Table 1.1, with a suggestion that only 1–2 per cent of people with Type 1 diabetes would need insulin pumps to manage their diabetes. Also, the therapy is not recommended at all for people with Type 2 diabetes, although small numbers of people with Type 2 diabetes use this therapy. Most of those with Type 2 diabetes had their pump initiated prior to NICE guidance being available, and anecdotally it has helped to manage severe insulin resistance.

In light of the information in the previous section of this chapter, the original NICE guidance (2003) was a large underestimation of the number of people who could benefit from this type of therapy, if the United Kingdom follows the lead from other countries, which is likely as more health professionals become confident and competent in using this therapy.

It is widely recognised that a great deal more research is required into insulin pump therapy, but it is likely to be a cost-effective treatment when measured

**Table 1.1**   Summary of 2003 NICE guidance on the use of insulin pump therapy

Insulin pump therapy is recommended in Type 1 diabetes only, where multiple-dose insulin (MDI) therapy, including using glargine* where appropriate, has failed. People using insulin pumps
should have the commitment and competence to use the therapy. The initiation should be carried out by a trained specialist team, usually a physician, diabetes specialist nurse and dietitian. There should be specific training provided for the pump user, ongoing support and a common core of advice agreed by the specialist team. Pumps can also be used in pregnancy and in children with diabetes.

*Definitions:*

• Failure of MDI therapy: when someone is unable to achieve HbA1c levels below 7.5% without disabling hypoglycaemia. If microalbuminuria or adverse features of the metabolic syndrome are present, the target level of HbA1c is lowered to below 6.5%.
• Disabling hypoglycaemia: repeated and unpredictable occurrence of hypoglycaemia requiring third-party assistance and causing continuing anxiety.

*Glargine was the only long-acting insulin analogue available at the time of publication of the guidance, and substitution of other long-acting analogues prior to using pump therapy is likely to have similar effects

against the cost of hospital admissions, the treatment of complications and time lost from work due to acute diabetes-related situations. Research indicates that the immediate financial savings, even without the reduction in long-term costs, are likely to make insulin pump therapy a cost-effective treatment (Ulahannan *et al.*, 2007). Quality of life is also a major consideration, with some studies reporting major improvements in many aspects (Hoogma *et al.*, 2005), but again further research is needed in this area. Chapter Three outlines some of the benefits that pump users perceive they have gained.

## WHAT WILL THE FUTURE LOOK LIKE?

Current technological advances in insulin pump therapy and glucose monitoring systems indicate that this type of therapy will become increasingly sophisticated over the next decade. Many of the devices that are currently being researched, together with others available in some parts of the world, are discussed in this section. Some of these devices have been available for a number of years but have failed to meet expectations, mainly because of safety reasons, but newer models might be developed to overcome these difficulties.

### Smaller pumps

One of the factors influencing pump choice for many pump users is the size of the pump they are going to use, with a preference for smaller models, and the manufacturers are being challenged to produce pumps that are smaller than their predecessors. While there are some essential features that all pumps require, such as an insulin reservoir, it is likely that newer and smaller models will emerge.

## Disposable devices

Disposable insulin pumps, developed in the United Kingdom, are a new innovation and are only now starting to be used. They have a reservoir of insulin and also a re-usable section that attaches to the skin, holds the battery and controls the flow of insulin. The pump user has a separate handheld programming device, rather than programming their insulin doses directly into the pump.

## Continuous glucose monitoring system linked to an insulin pump

Continuous glucose monitoring systems, which transmit data (wirelessly) to an insulin pump, are already available. The pump user inserts a second cannula, attached to a device known as a 'transmitter', that measures glucose levels in interstitial fluid and then converts the measurements to correlate with blood glucose levels. The result is displayed on the insulin pump, with information on whether the blood glucose is rising or falling and whether it is changing slowly or more rapidly. The pump can provide suggestions on insulin doses to give, based on the pump user programming their target blood glucose range and their usual bolus ratios.

These devices can be funded by the NHS, but it is more common for them to be purchased by pump users themselves, together with the disposable cannulae and sensors. Cost is one of the factors that limit the wider use of these devices, but other drawbacks include wearing two devices instead of one. Also, pump users still have to carry out fingerprick blood glucose readings to both calibrate the machine and to confirm their blood glucose levels prior to giving extra insulin doses, which might affect their perception of how much benefit will be gained from using such a device.

## Insulin delivery via a pre-inserted channel

Insulin can be infused directly into the peritoneum using a device implanted, under general anaesthetic, into the abdominal wall, with the pump tubing subsequently being attached. This method of insulin delivery has been available for a number of years and can help people with severe insulin resistance, as it bypasses subcutaneous tissue. It does, however, have a number of drawbacks, which include: a high risk of infections and blockage of the tubing, pain at the site of entry and crystallisation of the insulin. Also, because it is more intrusive, it carries a risk of causing psychological difficulties and altered body-image perceptions. For all these reasons, it is rarely used, is likely to remain in extremely limited use in its present form and is not currently initiated in the United Kingdom.

## Wireless insulin pumps

A wireless insulin pump that adheres to the skin as a patch, with an integral cannula, infusion set, insulin reservoir and battery, is available in the United States. It is changed every three days, and when it expires a new one is filled with insulin and applied. The programming of the pump and giving insulin doses is via a separate wireless device, which also has an integral blood glucose meter. One of the advantages of this device is that it does not have any tubing, so physical activity is made much easier, and also it does not have to be attached to clothing. This pump is not yet available in the United Kingdom.

## Implantable insulin pumps

Implantable insulin pumps were developed in the 1970s. They are inserted under general anaesthetic and carry a reservoir of U400 strength insulin, which is four times the strength of conventional U100 insulin used in the United Kingdom. The insulin lasts between one and two months before requiring a repeat operation to refill the reservoir. The pump user has a remote control to select their insulin dose. As with insulin delivery via a pre-inserted channel, the insulin is delivered into the abdomen, thereby reducing insulin resistance and enabling people to use lower doses of insulin. They also carry an increased risk of infections and blockages. The cost of these devices is high, and currently they are not used in the United Kingdom.

## Closed loop systems

A closed loop system of insulin delivery, where an insulin pump automatically delivers insulin at a variable rate in response to changing blood glucose levels, is often viewed as the gold standard in insulin pump therapy.

Ongoing research into this area shows promising results, but there are a number of challenges to overcome. The continuous glucose monitoring device used needs to be extremely accurate and of longer-lasting duration than those currently available, the device needs to be able to predict insulin requirements in the few minutes ahead and safety standards would need to be extremely high. It is likely to be a number of years before this type of device is available for general use.

## CONCLUSION

This chapter has provided an introduction to insulin pump therapy and an overview of the current situation in the United Kingdom, together with information about new devices under development and those that are available but in less common use. Information about the pumps currently used in the United Kingdom can be found in Chapter Four.

## REFERENCES

Diabetes Control and Complications Trial Research Group (1993) The effect of intensive treatment of diabetes on the development and progression of long-term complications in insulin-dependent diabetes mellitus. *New England Journal of Medicine* **329**(14): 977–986.

Diabetes UK (2006) Position statement: Insulin pump therapy, http://www.diabetes.org.uk/About_us/our_views/position_statements/insulin_pump_therapy, accessed 6 November 2007.

Everett J (2003) Insulin pump therapy: Where are we now? *Journal of Diabetes Nursing* **7**(6): 232–235.

Hoogma RPLM, Hammond PJ, Gomis R *et al.* (2005) Comparison of the effects of continuous subcutaneous insulin infusion (CSII) and NPH-based multiple daily insulin injections (MDI) on glycaemic control and quality of life: Results of the 5-nations trial. *Diabetic Medicine* **23**(2): 141–147.

National Institute for Health and Clinical Excellence (2003) *Guidance on the use of continuous subcutaneous insulin infusion for diabetes*, NICE, London.

Saudek CD (1997) Novel forms of insulin delivery. *Current Therapies for Diabetes* **26**(3): 599–610.

Teutsch SM, Herman WH, Dwyer DM *et al.* (1984) Mortality among diabetic patients using continuous subcutaneous insulin infusion pumps. *New England Journal of Medicine* **310**(6): 361–368.

Ulahannan T, Myint NN, Lonnen KF (2007) Making the case for insulin pump therapy. *Practical Diabetes International* **24**(5): 252–256.

Chapter 2
# The Advantages and Disadvantages of Insulin Pump Therapy

This chapter provides a broad outline of the main benefits, and the drawbacks, of insulin pump therapy. Some people who are considering a pump might feel negatively towards using an insulin pump initially but find that the benefits outweigh the disadvantages. Others might be enthusiastic but have not appreciated some of the more negative aspects. Both advantages and disadvantages should be fully discussed as part of a pre-pump assessment so that people can work out both the costs and the benefits to them as an individual and therefore make an informed decision about whether the therapy is right for them.

## THE ADVANTAGES OF INSULIN PUMP THERAPY

There is growing evidence in relation to some of the advantages of using insulin pump therapy, particularly when measuring medical parameters. For the benefits to individuals in relation to lifestyle, anecdotal evidence is more common, and more research is required into this area. This section discusses both the benefits identified in clinical trials and those seen in clinical practice.

## More physiological than other insulin regimens

Long-acting insulin analogues, developed in recent years, provide more stability than previously used isophane insulins, and NICE guidance (2003) suggests that analogues should be tried by people with Type 1 diabetes before being considered for insulin pump therapy. Long-acting analogue insulins reduce the risk of night-time hypoglycaemia in comparison to isophane insulin, and this contributes to stabilising blood glucose levels. However, pump users have the added advantage of being able to make very small adjustments to insulin doses, to successfully manage situations that would have been more difficult with multiple-dose insulin therapy, such as undertaking physical activity or controlling a dawn rise in their blood glucose levels. The small adjustments that can be made to insulin doses mean that physiological insulin production can be closely mimicked (Bolli, 1999).

## No more injections

Injecting insulin every day becomes a normal way of life for anyone with Type 1 diabetes and also for many with Type 2 diabetes. Anecdotally, many people say how much they would enjoy even a single day off from injecting. With a pump, there is still a need to insert a needle or cannula every two to three days, or sometimes more frequently, but the idea of no longer having to have insulin injections to regulate blood glucose levels is appealing to many people with diabetes and can be a strong reason why they wish to try pump therapy.

## Better glycaemic control

Studies looking specifically at glycaemic control suggest that a reduction in HbA1c of around 0.5 to 0.6 per cent can be gained from using insulin pump therapy rather than multiple daily injections (Pickup *et al.*, 2002), although those with a higher baseline HbA1c are likely to demonstrate a greater gain (Bode *et al.*, 1996). NICE guidance (2003) acknowledged that many clinical trials were conducted on people who had reasonable glycaemic control before entering the trial, and, in routine clinical practice, specialist teams report that much greater improvements in glycaemic control can be achieved (Everett, 2003).

## Reduced variation between individual blood glucose readings

While some might argue that the relatively small reduction in HbA1c suggests that the influence of pump therapy on glycaemic control is small, great benefit can be seen in the reduction in variation between individual blood glucose level readings across the day (Wredling *et al.*, 1997; Pickup *et al.*, 2002). Many people report feeling much better as a result of this, with comments such as: 'I didn't realise how awful I was feeling before I started using a pump – now I feel "normal" again!' The difference is also seen by relatives, and comments often include how more stable blood glucose levels have reduced mood swings:

'He's much easier to live with now' – or, from a parent – 'I feel like I've got my daughter back again; this is how she used to be.'

## Less hypoglycaemia

Recurrent hypoglycaemia, particularly with the loss of early-warning signs, is a common reason why someone might start to use an insulin pump. With injection therapy, the longer-acting insulin continues to work during the day and night, and can contribute to hypoglycaemia, particularly if someone undertakes vigorous physical activity. Because insulin doses can be finely tuned, many studies report a reduction in the amount of hypoglycaemia experienced by individuals using pumps (Bruttomesso *et al.*, 2002; Weissberg-Benchell *et al.*, 2003; Bode *et al.*, 1996). If people regularly experience severe hypoglycaemia – defined as requiring help from a third party rather than being able to recognise and treat it themselves – they experience even greater benefits when changing to using an insulin pump. They can also act promptly to reduce the basal insulin if required when hypoglycaemia occurs, to prevent further episodes.

## Improvement in complication-related symptoms

Using insulin pump therapy in people with severe symptomatic complications has been observed in clinical practice to reduce many of their symptoms, which is likely to be related to the reduction in variability between individual blood glucose readings and also better glycaemic control overall, although research is needed to confirm these findings. Examples include people with gastroparesis who require less frequent admissions to hospital because of their condition improving and those who have painful peripheral neuropathy, the symptoms of which have been reduced through using an insulin pump. This suggests that people beginning to develop complications might benefit from using insulin pumps, although this is not currently an indication for using a pump.

## Increased energy

Prior to using a pump, people often experience frequent hyperglycaemia, hypoglycaemia and large fluctuations in their blood glucose levels. Through using an insulin pump to closely match their body's requirements, anecdotally many pump users report feeling much more energetic and less lethargic.

Parents often report that their children seem more alert, and others report simple changes, such as finding it much easier to wake up in the morning.

## Food flexibility

To some extent, the introduction of Type 1 structured education programmes such as DAFNE (Dose Adjustment For Normal Eating) has enabled individuals to be more flexible using multiple-dose insulin therapy (Shearer *et al.*, 2004), but there are still some limitations to this flexibility. An insulin pump can give people a feeling of normality, of being able to do what others do, such as eating out or enjoying impromptu celebrations, and for some the enormous flexibility around what and when they eat is one of the key attractions (Bruttomesso *et al.*, 2002). A 45-year-old starting to use a pump, who had had diabetes since he was seven years old, remarked: 'It was the first time since I'd been diagnosed that I didn't *have* to eat to keep up with my insulin.'

## No long-acting insulin

Insulin pumps use short-acting insulin only. They can be used with soluble insulins, but most people use a rapid-acting insulin analogue (insulin lispro, insulin aspart or insulin glulisine) to enable them to make instant decisions about their insulin doses. Traditional long-acting insulins, such as isophane, have variable absorption rates of between 10 and 50 per cent per day (Lauritzen *et al.*, 1983), which accounts for some of the day-to-day variations in blood glucose levels that can occur. Although the newer long-acting insulin analogues have a more constant mode of action (Lepore *et al.*, 2000), it is not possible to stop or reduce the dose once they have been injected. Using only a rapid-acting analogue in a pump means that doses can be altered more confidently to deal with immediate situations, with a more reliable prediction of what effect the altered insulin dose will have on blood glucose levels.

## Easier to manage physical activity

Because of the lack of long-acting insulin, physical activity is easier to manage, as the pump user can alter their insulin doses easily rather than have to eat large amounts of carbohydrate. Background or basal insulin rates can be reduced, or the pump can be removed for a short time if preferred, particularly for activities such as contact sports. Following activity, both basal and bolus doses can be reduced if necessary, in order to avoid delayed hypoglycaemia caused by the body replacing its glycogen stores.

## Sleeping in

Having a leisurely start to the day becomes much easier using pump therapy, as it no longer matters what time breakfast is eaten – or even whether it is eaten at all. Many pump users report that they feel they have significantly more flexibility regarding their sleep patterns than they previously experienced when using injection therapy (Hoogma *et al.*, 2005). Basal rates can be set by the pump user to ensure they can stay in bed later and neither experience hypoglycaemia nor wake with a high blood glucose level.

## Reduced insulin doses

Many people report that they require a significantly smaller amount of insulin over a 24-hour period, because they are taking precisely the insulin dose they require. When someone starts to use an insulin pump, initially their pre-pump total daily insulin dose will be decreased by 30 per cent or more. Individuals will vary regarding how much insulin they need to re-introduce to stabilise their blood glucose level, but an average reduction of around 14 per cent has been found in clinical trials (Pickup *et al.*, 2002), which still brings the total to less than prior to using a pump.

## Easier weight management

Using multiple-dose insulin therapy can make it difficult to manage weight, in particular to lose weight, because it is hard to adjust insulin doses precisely enough to match a reduction in food intake. People trying to lose weight might also want to undertake additional physical activity, which, when combined with less food, can result in hypoglycaemia. The preciseness with which insulin doses can be matched to food intake and physical activity can be of great benefit to pump users wishing to lose weight.

## Regaining personal confidence

People who experience regular or unpredictable hypoglycaemia might become less confident or depressed through dealing with life and their diabetes on a day-to-day basis. They might feel unable to join in spontaneous activities or social events, preferring to stick to a more rigid routine to try and maintain their glycaemic control or avoid suffering the embarrassment of a hypoglycaemic episode in public. For these people, using an insulin pump can be a way of regaining confidence that their insulin treatment can be more reliable and predictable. Pump users report feeling able to socialise more, getting new jobs and developing their careers, being more outgoing and generally feeling much happier with their lives. In studies incorporating quality-of-life measures, pump users report a significant decrease in aspects such as 'diabetes-related worry', and also indicate that diabetes has less of an impact on their daily lives (Hoogma *et al.*, 2005; Bruttomesso *et al.*, 2002).

## Summary

All the above are the main benefits that are related to the use of insulin pump therapy, from research studies and also reported by pump users. This list of benefits is not exhaustive, and the varied experiences of individuals are likely to demonstrate a far wider range of benefits from their point of view. Identifying the benefits that exist for each person can help in setting realistic targets, for example reducing the frequency of hypoglycaemic episodes could be the main aim for one person, while for another it might be to have less time off work for diabetes-related illnesses.

## THE DISADVANTAGES OF INSULIN PUMP THERAPY

As with any type of treatment, there are some disadvantages to using insulin pump therapy, and, despite some people with diabetes seeing the benefits of using a pump, these might be outweighed for them by one or more of the disadvantages listed below. For these people, even if the benefits of insulin pump therapy seem clear, it is unlikely to be a solution. This section discusses the main drawbacks to pump use for individuals.

## Need to wear the pump continuously

While it is possible to remove an insulin pump for a short while, for example while showering, swimming or engaging in short periods of physical activity, it needs to be worn for the majority of every 24-hour period to realise the potential benefit of improved glycaemic control. Many pump users have no issue with this and see it as no more inconvenient than carrying a mobile phone or pager. For a minority, it is a major issue, viewed as an unwelcome intrusion, a physical and constant reminder of their diabetes or as an alteration of their body image. For these people, pump use is unlikely to be successful, no matter what improvements could be gained in glycaemic control.

## Inability to 'think like a pancreas'

Insulin pumps are a technological tool that are sometimes described as being able to 'think like a pancreas', giving the misleading impression that the pump user can simply attach the pump and then forget about their diabetes. Currently, although some pumps are able to provide suggestions regarding what insulin dose is required, no pumps will automatically alter the insulin doses being infused, and potential pump users should be made aware that pumps will only carry out the functions they are programmed to by the pump user themselves.

## More proactive management required

The success of an insulin pump is based not only on reliable, sophisticated technology but also on what the pump user does with it. It is important not to underestimate or minimise the amount of hard work and decision-making that is involved with managing an insulin pump. Regular blood glucose testing, calculating bolus doses, altering basal rates and reviewing the success of actions taken are a daily part of managing insulin pump therapy. For some people with diabetes, this might be no more onerous than their management of multiple-dose insulin therapy, but others might find the amount of work to be too much, and prefer to continue with injection therapy.

## Psychological impact

The potential negative psychological impact of wearing a pump can play a major part in deciding whether it is the right therapy for an individual. As mentioned above, this constant reminder of diabetes can be resented, and it makes it difficult for people who want to 'simply inject and then get on with life' to choose this type of therapy. Feeling the pump is on show to others and being apprehensive about its potential effect on both social and sexual relationships can be reasons why some individuals choose not to use insulin pump therapy, or who try it and then discontinue it after a brief period.

It is important to explore these issues with someone, and to offer further psychological help or support if appropriate, as they might be indicators of a deeper dissatisfaction in relation to their diabetes. Some might not wish to explore it further but simply accept that the burden of wearing a pump is too much for them. They might make comments such as 'I know it will be good for my diabetes, but I just don't want to wear it' or 'I can see the benefits, but it's not for me just now'. Accepting how the individual feels, rather than adopting a persuasive attitude, leaves the door open for future discussion, when the person might feel more positive towards insulin pump therapy.

## CONCLUSION

This chapter has outlined the main advantages and disadvantages of insulin pump use and highlighted the need for full discussions with people prior to using a pump, to find out their expectations and ensure they understand what it entails. The huge benefits that can be gained from the therapy might be overshadowed for some people with diabetes by the drawbacks, and ultimately pump users need to be committed to using the therapy effectively. More information about many of the aspects discussed in this chapter can be found throughout the rest of this book.

## REFERENCES

Bode BMW, Steed RD, Davidson PC (1996) Reduction in severe hypoglycemia with long-term continuous subcutaneous insulin infusion in type 1 diabetes. *Diabetes Care* **19**(4): 324–327.

Bolli GB (1999) How to ameliorate the problem of hypoglycaemia in intensive as well as non intensive treatment of type 1 diabetes. *Diabetes Care* **22**(suppl. 2): B43–B52.

Bruttomesso D, Pianta A, Crazzolara D *et al.* (2002) Continuous subcutaneous insulin infusion (CSII) in the Veneto region: Efficacy, acceptability and quality of life. *Diabetic Medicine* **19**(8): 628–634.

Everett J (2003) Insulin pump therapy: Where are we now? *Journal of Diabetes Nursing* **7**(6): 232–235.

Hoogma RPLM, Hammond PJ, Gomis R *et al.* (2005) Comparison of the effects of continuous subcutaneous insulin infusion (CSII) and NPH-based multiple daily insulin injections (MDI) on glycaemic control and quality of life: Results of the 5-nations trial. *Diabetic Medicine* **23**(2): 141–147.

Lauritzen T, Pramming S, Deckert T, Binder C (1983) Pharmacokinetics of continuous subcutaneous insulin infusion. *Diabetologia* **24**(5): 326–329.

Lepore M, Pampanelli S, Fanelli C *et al.* (2000) Pharmacokinetics and pharmacodynamics of subcutaneous injection of long-acting human insulin analog glargine, NPH insulin and ultralente human insulin and continuous subcutaneous infusion of insulin lispro. *Diabetes* **49**: 2142–2148.

National Institute for Health and Clinical Excellence (2003) *Guidance on the use of continuous subcutaneous insulin infusion for diabetes*, NICE, London.

Pickup J, Mattock M, Kerry S (2002) Glycaemic control with continuous subcutaneous insulin infusion compared with intensive insulin injections in patients with type 1 diabetes: Meta-analysis of randomised controlled trials. *British Medical Journal* **324**(7339): 705–708.

Shearer A, Bagust A, Sanderson D *et al.* (2004) Cost-effectiveness of flexible intensive insulin management to enable dietary freedom in people with Type 1 diabetes in the UK. *Diabetic Medicine* **21**(5): 460–467.

Weissberg-Benchell J, Antisdel-Lomaglio J, Seshadri R (2003) Insulin pump therapy: A meta-analysis. *Diabetes Care* **26**(4): 1079–1087.

Wredling R, Hannerz L, Johansson U-B (1997) Variability of blood glucose levels in patients treated with continuous subcutaneous insulin infusion: A pilot study. *Practical Diabetes International* **14**(1): 5–8.

# Chapter 3
# The Experiences of Insulin Pump Users

Whether a pump will benefit someone is often looked at by health professionals from a clinical point of view – whether it is likely to help the particular situation, and also whether the local agreements about pumps, including guidelines, selection criteria and funding, will support its use. From the perspective of someone with diabetes, the view can be very different. During the course of writing this book, one of the comments made by a pump user was: 'Professionals dealing with pump users need to be aware of what a big step it is for someone to go onto a pump', and while there is some awareness of this, hearing their perspective can be enlightening and helpful.

This chapter uses narratives and experiences from a wide range of people with diabetes, including those using pumps, those who are contemplating using pumps and those who have decided that a pump is not for them. It will help raise awareness of the thoughts and feelings experienced by many people starting pump therapy, what they have found helpful in the care they have received and their views on some aspects of pump therapy management. However, no two people are alike, and it is important not to prejudge or assume that we know what fears or concerns people have. Finding out what potential pump users really think through having honest, non-judgemental conversations with them will mean that decisions are made on an informed basis and with awareness on both sides.

## DISCUSSING INSULIN PUMPS IN CONSULTATIONS

With the limited availability of funding for insulin pumps, inequality in service provision across the country and also variable enthusiasm and expertise on the part of health professionals, approaches to discussing insulin pumps with people with diabetes can vary enormously from one diabetes team to another. In some, the suitability of an insulin pump might be discussed by health professionals as a good treatment option, but in a lot of situations people with diabetes are the ones who initially raise the topic of whether an insulin pump might be available for them, and often believe that it is unlikely to be available because of the lack of NHS funding:

> A friend who works for NHS Direct suggested to me that an insulin pump might help (at the time I was spending as much time in A & E with hypos as I was at home and would have tried anything). I asked my diabetes team and was surprised to find they agreed straight away, and were even already thinking about it as an option, which caught me off guard. I was expecting a bit more of an argument.
>
> I have friends who use pumps, and they look so well and tell me how their HbA1c is much better. One of them always looked pale and about to pass out and now feels great. It had been something I had thought about and was positive about, but thought, due to the lack of funding, it wouldn't happen.
>
> I initiated discussions about getting a pump as I'd read a report on them and found out that the clinic was getting some.

For some, discussions about pumps are not such a good experience:

> The last time I was at the hospital, I was told that a pump might be considered as a last resort for me, as everything else had been tried. I was also informed that I would need to be assessed regarding whether I was an acceptable candidate, and that if it didn't work I would be taken off it. I had felt positive about pumps before this, but the way it was portrayed was scary.
>
> I asked about an insulin pump at my diabetes clinic but was told that it wasn't the right treatment for me, that they are very complicated and that a lot of things could go wrong with them.

Also, even when funding appears to have been approved, in reality experiences are not always positive:

> I was expecting to get a pump in May, and contacted the clinic to find out what dates my training would be, but then was told the clinic weren't getting as many as they thought so I couldn't have one. I was devastated, not least by the manner I had found out, almost by accident, that I was not getting one. In the end, I had to wait over a year before I got my pump.

While the inequality of insulin pump use across the country might take many years to be redressed, it is important that people be given realistic information in clinics. The myths of pumps being dangerous, likely to malfunction and cause ketoacidosis, and that they should not be used unless all else has failed, are unfounded, as can be seen in Chapter One. Providing people with information about insulin pumps, where they can find out more (particularly if the diabetes team have limited expertise) and making sure they have their questions answered should be the first steps for anyone enquiring about pumps. Finding out what they already know and supplementing this information, including dispelling any myths they might hold, are ways to start holding useful conversations about whether a pump is the best option or not for them. Also, having agreements locally about funding for insulin pumps, as discussed in Chapter Five, will help to ensure that realistic conversations are held with people regarding whether an insulin pump is likely to be available for them.

## THOUGHTS AND CONCERNS ABOUT PUMP USE

Even if someone is enthusiastic about starting to use an insulin pump, and feels it is the best option for their diabetes, it can still cause a lot of anxiety. They might have had many years of experience with injecting, which, even if it is not achieving optimal glycaemic control, is a system they are familiar with and used to managing. Apprehension is common:

> I felt in control before, in charge, and didn't want to be a beginner again, so I resisted it initially.
>
> I was terrified and excited about getting my pump – terrified of the unknown and also of the possibility that it wouldn't be the answer I hoped for. Excited at something new after 20 years of diabetes, and at the prospect of good control with fewer hypos.
>
> I felt apprehensive initially – I felt I would be less in control of what was happening.
>
> Apart from the physical worries, my other concern was that if I tried the pump and didn't like it I'd be stuck with it, as having waited so long for it I couldn't then reject it!

For some, the emotions are even stronger, and many people reflect on their diabetes as a whole, often facing up to thoughts and feelings that they have not confronted prior to this time:

> The pump was verbally offered as a last resort. It made me panic and, for something that I thought I desperately wanted, I found myself not wanting it at all, which was hard to come to terms with. The regimen I had didn't work, but if the pump didn't work I'd have to go back on a system that has been proven to not work.

Having discussions about the pump, I confessed to my boyfriend for probably the first time that my diabetes wasn't all that it seemed and that it never had been. Being honest with him, I was being honest with myself: my diabetes is a mess, it's not a phase, it won't get better, I'm not just going to wake up one day and like magic I'll start to follow the textbook on diabetes.

People also have many and varied questions, even at an early stage, and need to find answers to be able to make an informed choice about whether they feel they want an insulin pump or will be able to manage it:

I was worried about being permanently attached to a machine.

It is daunting even if you are keen, and doubly so for patients for whom the pump is the last resort, and who might feel that they are being forced into getting one.

This 'alarming' is a big concern to me: what if I take it off, have a shower, forget about it and go to work and it alarms in the house while I am 22 miles away? Or worse still, it alarms and I'm at work, what do I do then? Or does this mean that not only am I attached to the pump but I have to carry a kitbag full of medical stuff just in case?

I was worried it would suddenly take over my life: that pen over there is the diabetic side of me, but isn't attached to me, but a pump would be. I would be the freak with the pump.

What if I wanted a day off? With injections, when all else fails, you can just have a 'day off' from your diabetes. This is when all around you is falling apart and you feel so out of control. By having a 'day off', you can still feel in control, even though that means your diabetes is out of control. What if you decided to do that if you were using a pump?

What about if you get old, become infirm or can't see, do you get taken off the pump?

What of holidays? I've never been a one for a bikini but still where do you put the pump? I suppose a swim in the ocean is out of the question and what about sweat/sunbathing/suncream?

Do I end up with track marks over my stomach? Will I end up with a bigger stomach as it's in there all the time?

These comments from people with diabetes provide a small insight into the worries that people might have, from leaving behind a system where they felt in control even though their blood glucose levels might not have been ideal to worrying about how big an impact the pump would have on their lives, and also many queries about how to deal with day-to-day situations. Unanswered questions can cause increased anxiety and stress, so helping people with diabetes find answers to their questions is an important part of helping someone who might be considering using pump therapy.

It is also possible to wrongly anticipate the concerns that people might have about pumps, or whether they will be able to put the additional work in to make it a success. For example, in the insulin pump trials in the United Kingdom in the 1990s, health professionals were surprised that people choosing to enter the trial did not seem worried about wearing the pump 24 hours a day, counting carbohydrates and testing their blood glucose levels at least four times a day.

> I was told that the only downfall was the fact I would have to test my blood more often than I was doing, but that's a small price to pay for better control.

In recent years, the introduction of structured education programmes for people with Type 1 diabetes across the country has placed a stronger focus on a more active management of the condition, so changing from injection therapy to pump therapy might involve fewer changes than previously for some. As already discussed, it is important to be clear about how much work is involved in pump therapy so that people can make an informed choice about whether they wish to proceed.

## BODY IMAGE AND RELATIONSHIPS

Being attached to a pump 24 hours a day can cause anxiety for some, although others might feel less self-conscious. For those who have major concerns, discussion might help, but feelings like these can put some people off pump therapy despite the beneficial effect it can have on blood glucose levels:

> I know the consultant wants me to use a pump, and the past 24 hours of using a pump has already shown me that it can help my diabetes, but I hate it. I just cried all night. I feel it's a big intrusion in my life and I can't cope with it.
>
> I might think about a pump when I'm in a stable relationship, but I just can't imagine how I would explain it to a new boyfriend. I'm worried it will make me feel less sexy.
>
> Wearing a pump is like wearing a big neon sign stating: 'Warning: diabetic!' I'm just me, who just happens to need to inject before they eat. I have a pen. The pen is separate from me. I take it with me when needed and leave it behind when I don't. That is the separate diabetic bit of me.

It can also have an effect on relationships, and pump users report that it is much easier if they are already in an established relationship than if they are single and hoping to meet the right person:

> All I could think was of all those intimate moments that would now be ruined by a piece of kit attached to me.
>
> I have quite a few nice dresses, so what was I to do now? A slinky dress worn with a bulge or looking like I have three boobs?
>
> What about the needle thing that goes in you with an Opsite-type dressing on your body – how attractive must that look?
>
> What if my boyfriend was to knock it or pull it out in his sleep for instance and then for hours I had no insulin going round my system? What if he was frightened to come near me in case he harmed me or broke the pump?
>
> Imagine having eaten and then putting a hand down your front to remove the pump so you can alter how much insulin is going in. Oh how romantic!

However, even in a stable relationship, partners and close family can have negative views about whether an insulin pump is a good idea:

> My husband was not convinced that it was worth it and felt that the pump would get in the way and make my diabetes more intrusive.
>
> My daughter got very distressed when she saw the pump and kept crying and trying to pull it off me. I ended up feeling it wasn't safe to use the pump just now. Maybe I'll try it again when she's a bit older.

Encouraging people to express their worries about wearing the pump, and also the effect it will have on close relationships, will help people reflect on their own situations and be realistic about whether the impact of wearing a pump will be positive or negative. If issues are not discussed fully, there is a greater chance of the person with diabetes only wearing the pump for a short period before deciding to revert back to injections. Close family, or people that the pump user feels are important to them, should be encouraged to attend appointments, to ask questions and to have their own concerns addressed, as their views are likely to play a major part in whether pump therapy is the right choice for them and also whether it will succeed.

## EARLY DAYS WITH PUMP THERAPY

Many people who use insulin pumps report high levels of anxiety in the early days of using a pump. They are faced with technology that is new to them, and are also often confronting major fears when trying to manage their diabetes in a different way, fears that have built up over many years of experience of using injection therapy:

> The pump training itself was good but also quite overwhelming as there is so much to learn.
>
> It's like relearning about diabetes, going back to basics again.
>
> You have to believe in the pump and that you're not going to go hypo all the time, which is scary when you're used to just blacking out.
>
> I felt really ignorant, starting out with a new system, and uncertain about whether I was making the right decisions about my insulin doses.

Support from health professionals is crucial, which can be provided by developing a system that has easy access when required, but also encourages the pump user to experiment and start to make their own decisions:

> Initially, you have a lot of questions and need a great deal of support both face to face and on the phone.
>
> The manufacturer's helpline is useful, but there are times when you need to speak to someone who knows you and is aware of your individual needs. My diabetes nurse gave me her mobile phone number, which made me feel more secure and ensured I was always able to contact someone should an emergency occur.
>
> I found the user manual wasn't very helpful: some of the information was so confusing, I couldn't work it out without the help of my diabetes nurse.

Many people also report that knowing other pump users is helpful, and developing systems that encourage interaction and sharing ideas, including what hasn't worked for them, helps people feel more confident in starting to make their own decisions:

> I was fortunate as my diabetes nurse had arranged for two of us to start the pumps together, so we both supported each other on the day and subsequently.
>
> I think that, where possible and if everyone agrees, starting two or more people on the pump at the same time allows you to meet people in your position and hopefully find another means of support in the early days. I have been asked to set up a pump users' support group locally and again think this is a good way to help people help and support themselves.
>
> One useful thing was to attend a Diabetes UK meeting where there were two people on pumps, one who had been on one for four days, the other for four years, and to hear their experiences. I also was able to email a friend of mine with some of my worries and concerns, and she was able to answer my questions and help me that way.

Ensuring that an adequate amount of support is available in the early days is important, and Chapter Five discusses in more detail how that might be achieved within a specialist service. Helping provide opportunities to meet others in similar situations, and creating time for them to share and compare their experiences, has also been shown here to be valuable, and should be built into service provision where possible.

## ONGOING MANAGEMENT OF THE PUMP

As pump users become more experienced, they find ways of dealing with different situations that work best for them. For example, there are many different ways of giving either a larger or a smaller dose of insulin, such as starting and stopping the pump, using temporary basal rates and using different types of bolus. The general approach to education should be to help people understand how the pump delivers insulin and then helping them apply that to the day-to-day situations they find themselves in. The following quotes show the wide variety of day-to-day issues that people deal with and how they have managed to find success through experimenting with their insulin pump.

At work, I have an hour of a lot of activity and then it depends if it's busy. If we have a lot of customers, I spend the day mainly talking; if it's quiet, I might spend all day polishing the cars, which makes me hypo. So I've set two different basal rates, one for the busy days and one for the quiet days, and I can just switch them over when I need to.

Being able to change insulin to carbohydrate ratios and basal rates for different times of day allows you great flexibility and accuracy. I have had a lot less hypos, and those I have had have been much less pronounced and have required much less treatment to correct them.

Going to the gym is much easier as I can reduce my basal rate temporarily, and for the first time ever I have been able to avoid post-exercise hypos and the need for excessive calorie intake!

I think the pump is great, but every day, after my shower, I just sit and have 30 minutes without it, just to make me feel normal, then I'm happy to wear it the rest of the day.

In the early days, I got a bit complacent, and for one evening meal I got the figures wrong – I thought each item had 15 grams of carbohydrate in, but it should have been 15 grams per 100 grams. I had a major hypo, just as bad as I used to, but it helped me to look more closely at what I was eating.

When you go out for a meal, you don't know how the meal has been prepared or what has been used in the cooking, so calculating the carbohydrate content is not easy. Now I'm more used to it, I can give a good guess as to how much is in most meals and, if I'm wrong, just put it right later.

It took a while to get used to positioning the cannula and sticking the tape down with only two hands, and when I used the left or right side of my body, I found it hard to see, reach and of course get it correct.

Sometimes it takes a lot of confidence to give the amount of insulin that is needed; sometimes I feel it's easier to run my blood sugars a bit higher, but then I see my HbA1c creeping up and have to work harder at it again.

These scenarios show that people often put in a lot of hard work and spend a lot of time thinking and planning how they can manage their pump therapy. They also show that sometimes complacency can set in, but people learn the most from experience and through making their own mistakes. Encouraging discussion of how they have managed different situations, what has worked, what hasn't worked and what they will do in the same situation in the future helps build up their decision-making and coping skills and helps them apply their existing knowledge to new situations.

## USING COMPUTER-GENERATED DATA

The majority of insulin pumps have a download facility that enables pump users to transfer the data in their pump to a computer and analyse it, alongside their downloaded blood glucose readings, to identify trends and work out where changes need to be made. Whether someone finds this useful can depend on their own understanding of the data, their perception of whether they feel it is useful and how they choose to manage their pump therapy. Some people feel very positively about using this type of program, particularly in relation to blood glucose results:

Downloading results from my meter helps me look at trends of blood glucose to identify problem areas that need addressing. Without this technology, I would find myself reacting to individual glucose readings rather than taking a proactive approach to my glycaemic control.

I personally find that being able to see the readings converted into a chart or graph is far easier for me to understand than looking at a load of numbers. They help you to spot trends in your readings for carbs, insulin dose and illness, and I feel this is a real benefit as you have a chance of staying one step ahead and reducing the problems before they hit.

Keeping up to date with developments in technology and learning how to use them effectively to help me get the right balance has been an important part of my life with diabetes. I now use structured blood glucose self-testing and computer downloading of the results to help me get the most from my insulin pump therapy.

However, not everyone has the same view:

> I'm sure the computer download can be useful if you like computers and if the information helps you make choices that you otherwise might not have seen. However, I don't use it – probably too lazy! – but also I try not to analyse things too much or make diabetes my hobby.
>
> Blood testing results are useful, but it's a lot of work to get much use from them, and I don't download consistently enough to learn a great deal.
>
> I find there are downsides to the programs I use: you can't set the times of meals to the trend that you use. They work on a default scale and you must remember to go in and check the settings before you download or some normal readings are marked as too high or too low. Also, the daily data list prints with your last test result at the top, so you have to read it backwards, in effect.
>
> The rep gave me a cable to let me download my pump data but didn't explain what to do with the results or what they meant. She was meant to come back to me but didn't, so although I've downloaded the data and looked at all the pretty graphs they haven't been much use to me!

Helping people to understand the software they have, and how the downloaded data can be used to manage the pump, will equip people with enough knowledge to decide whether they want to use it as part of managing their pump therapy. As has been shown, it might be either embraced or rejected, and it is important to allow people to make their own decisions, rather than trying to use the computer program to please their health professional. Helping people find the most useful system to review their progress that works for them is more likely to result in their proactively managing pump therapy.

## OVERALL PERCEPTIONS

It is important to remember that not everything about using a pump is positive, and some aspects can be more difficult. Also, pump users need to be prepared to manage their pump well, even at the times when diabetes is not their first priority:

> You have to remember that you have a pump, because if you don't then you can very easily catch it and pull the tube, which might make the cannula move and so you have to check your blood more frequently.

You can't just jump under a shower without sorting your pump out first, and that can be extremely frustrating when you're feeling sweaty or dirty.

You need to do a lot of tests to check how things are working, although I did a lot anyway and I'm sure the number will reduce.

There is a lot to learn, and so you need to be very motivated and take on board a lot of information if you are going to gain the full benefits.

Going to the toilet can be interesting – with the short tubes, you need to find somewhere to put the pump. Also, if you go out for the day, not all public toilets have a place to put your pump while you use the loo.

I couldn't wait to get rid of my pump. It just felt like diabetes was taking over my life. I felt I was always testing and was beginning to feel depressed.

Despite the difficulties, with adequate discussion before changing from injection therapy, most people choose to continue using their pump and feel that it gives them a great many advantages that were not there when using injection therapy:

The main advantage for me is freedom! Not having to inject at night time is strangely liberating.

Within a week, I had decided that I would not give my pump up for any reason! I also wished that I'd had the opportunity to have a pump years ago, although I realise that the state-of-the-art pump I have now was not around even a couple of years ago.

It can change your life for the better in so many ways but you do have to be committed and be prepared to work hard. The first week or so you might well want to give up, but get past that and you'll never want to be without one!

The main advantage the pump has given me is the confidence to start doing things again without the fear of hypos. I feel so much better that it has given me a whole new lease of life. I feel that I can now do things that I would not even have considered before getting the pump.

I feel that the pump has made so much of a difference that it's hard to list how it's affected my life.

I feel normal for the first time since I was diagnosed. I didn't realise how unwell I felt up to now.

I have always felt diabetes was the enemy and that everything was a battle, but now it's much more of a partnership.

I used to hate testing my blood sugar, but now it's great. Most of the results are good ones, but if I get one that's too high or too low now I can do something about it. I feel in control again.

I used to wake up feeling like I had a hangover every day, but now I feel full of energy.

When I was in a bad mood, everyone always blamed my diabetes and didn't take me seriously. Now, when I'm in a bad mood, it's just because I am, not because I'm having a hypo.

After 10 years of diabetes, I feel I've got my son back. He's so much easier to live with now.

How people feel about their pump is likely to be reflected in how they manage it, and pumps can be a source of anxiety and depression for some, and seem like a miracle to others. Opportunities should exist within clinics for pump users to talk about how they feel about their pump and to share experiences with others, and, at any time, they should be able to revert to injection therapy, either temporarily or permanently, if they believe it is the right decision for them.

## CONCLUSION

This chapter has provided a snapshot of the experiences of some pump users, both positive and negative. Having open and honest discussions with them, and finding out what their anxieties are about using a pump, will increase the chances of pump therapy being a success if it is the type of therapy chosen. Providing adequate support in the early days has been shown to be important, as is giving people opportunities to talk about their day-to-day management, both their successes and those things that have worked less well, not only with health professionals but also with other pump users. The pros and cons of using pumps, even for those who are keen, are summarised in this quote:

Changing to a pump has been one of the most profound experiences of my life. I took care of my diabetes before, and technology has made it easier in one way, but in another there's more potential for me to get obsessed with it, and never stop thinking about having diabetes.

Finally, pumps are not for everyone, and if someone is struggling to manage with a pump, or is finding that their quality of life is worse than when using injections, discontinuing pump therapy is likely to help them be able to cope better with managing their diabetes.

# Chapter 4
# Insulin Pumps and Infusion Sets

There are a number of different companies that manufacture pumps which are available in the United Kingdom. The pumps have a number of generic features and functions, and some also have additional features and functions that can be useful. There are similarities in price between pumps produced by different companies, although some pumps with special features tend to be more expensive. This chapter will discuss the types of features that pumps have, and will also provide information on infusion sets, including their similarities and differences. For more detailed information on any pump or infusion set, the manufacturer should be contacted.

## GENERAL FEATURES OF INSULIN PUMPS

There are a number of insulin pump functions that are common to most pumps, although the method of programming and the use of these functions will vary from one model or manufacturer to another. This section discusses each function in turn, and how they might be put into practical use.

## Basal rates

An insulin pump infuses insulin continuously throughout the day and night, and the amounts of insulin it is programmed to deliver each hour are known collectively as the 'basal rate'. The basal rate can be programmed in either hourly or half-hourly increments, giving a total of either 24 or 48 periods that can be set at different doses if required. The lowest basal rates per hour vary between pumps from 0.025 units per hour to 0.1 units per hour, although much larger doses can be set if required.

To maintain good glycaemic control, the pump user is likely to need different basal rates at different times of the day, and the hourly or half-hourly rates are titrated over a period of days or weeks in response to blood glucose results, until the blood glucose levels are almost all within the individual's target range. As with injection therapy, it will never be possible to find a single basal rate that will be ideal over months or years, so pump users also have to regularly review their basal rates and make changes as required. Many pumps also have the option of programming more than one basal rate so that the pump user can switch to a different rate when required, for example when working different shifts. Depending on the type of pump used, the additional basal rates might need to be programmed directly into the pump, or alternatively a computer program can be used to set up a different basal rate, which can then be downloaded into the pump when it is needed.

Insulin pumps also have the capacity to deliver a temporary increase or reduction in the basal rate, for example someone might need only 50 per cent of their usual insulin dose if they are being particularly active for a couple of hours, or alternatively might need 150 per cent or more of their insulin dose if they are unwell. More information on how to set an initial basal rate, use different basal rate functions and titrate basal rates in relation to blood glucose levels can be found in Chapter 10.

## Bolus features

A 'bolus dose' is the term used for an additional insulin dose that can be given at any time, usually to either match carbohydrate intake or to correct a high blood glucose level. There are three types of bolus, which vary in how the insulin is delivered, and also might be referred to by different names, depending on the manufacturer. The types of bolus, with the alternative names shown in brackets, are:

- Standard bolus (normal bolus): this is where the whole of the programmed dose is delivered immediately, within a few seconds of programming, in the same way as a subcutaneous injection would deliver insulin.
- Extended bolus (square wave): this is where a bolus dose of insulin is programmed into the pump and then delivered at a constant rate over a longer period, varying from a few minutes to a few hours. It is used in situations where the whole of the insulin is not required immediately, and pump users can select not only the dose but also the length of time over which they want the insulin to be delivered.
- Mixed bolus (multiwave, dual wave, combo): this is a combination of the first two boluses, where the pump is programmed to deliver part of the programmed dose immediately and part of it over a longer time period, and the pump user can choose how it is divided and over how long.

The choice of type of bolus to use normally depends on the type or amount of food being eaten. How to calculate what bolus amounts to give in relation to carbohydrate intake is discussed in Chapter Seven, and the use of the variety of bolus options in general is discussed in Chapter 10.

## Visual display

All pumps have a visual display, similar to that of a mobile phone, and also a backlight that can be activated to ensure the display is clearly visible. Most of the display screens go blank a number of seconds after the pump user has finished pressing any of the buttons, to save the battery. Some pumps have the option of programming the amount of time preferred before the display goes blank. The displays commonly show the amount of basal insulin being delivered at the time, and pressing buttons in specific sequences will take the pump user through the menu and allow them to select which function they would like to activate or alter. The same buttons are used, in sequence, to set the clock, alarms and other parameters, as well as infusion rates and additional doses of insulin to be delivered.

## Water resistance

The pumps are all tested for water resistance, and the manufacturers can provide information on how waterproof a specific model is. This rating applies to when the pumps leave the factory, but daily wear and tear can cause hairline cracks in the casing that have the potential to let water in. In general, most pumps will function correctly if they have been accidentally submerged in water and removed immediately, but they might need to be disconnected before undertaking swimming or watersports. Some companies produce waterproof covers that can be used, with instructions that need to be carefully followed to ensure the pump stays dry, although removal of the pump is still likely to be the safest option.

## Alarm functions

All the pumps have alarm systems as part of their safety features. Standard functions include alarms to indicate when the amount of insulin is getting low – most are set to alarm when 20 units of insulin are left, but some can be individually programmed, depending on the pump user's preference. Alarms also indicate when the battery is low, and the manufacturer's instructions will indicate how much battery life they are likely to have once the alarm has been activated, although changing the battery as soon as the alarm has been activated is recommended. Many of the pumps have additional alarms, for example to indicate when an occlusion has occurred and pressure has built up in the tubing or for customised settings. Some pumps also have the option of programming alarms as reminders, for example to test blood glucose levels a specific time after a meal. The handbook that accompanies a pump provides specific information on what action to take in the event of an alarm being activated.

## Audible beeps and vibrations

The pumps have a combination of audible beeps and vibrations, and the pump user can decide what operating mode they wish to keep their pump in. For example, some of the pumps beep whenever a button is pressed or give confirming beeps for the amount of bolus insulin being delivered. The audible beeps can be turned off and the pump can be set to vibrate only.

## Memory functions

All the pumps store data in their memories, with variations in the amount and type of information they store. Recent insulin doses can be looked up, which is helpful if someone is unsure whether they have given a bolus dose or not, and is highly appreciated by many pump users. Daily insulin dose totals, boluses given and the last alarms that were activated are examples of the type of information stored in the pump memory. Some pumps can also store blood glucose readings in their memory and can produce graphs showing trends of readings over a few hours or longer periods.

## Keylocks

All pumps have a keylock, similar to a mobile phone, to prevent any accidental altering of settings or giving extra insulin unintentionally. The keylock is activated by either pressing the buttons in sequence or entering a security code, and this stops the pump user – or anyone else – being able to access any of the functions. A sequence of buttons, or re-entering the security code, will deactivate the lock at any time. Using the keylock can provide reassurance to the pump user that their insulin doses cannot be tampered with, and also that when they are asleep accidental pressing of buttons will not result in extra doses of insulin being given. Parents of young children with insulin pumps also find the keylock function useful.

## FEATURES OF INDIVIDUAL PUMPS

As insulin pumps become increasingly sophisticated, many of them now have advanced features that can provide additional benefits, although the pump user still has the choice of using whichever functions they wish, and some will choose to only use the basic functions. This section will highlight the advanced features available with some pumps, and what advantages they have.

## Connection with a blood glucose sensor

Some pumps link wirelessly with a continuous glucose monitoring sensor (see Chapter One for more information on how this works). The sensor is worn for up to three days continuously, and it transmits blood glucose readings to the pump every five minutes, together with information about which direction the blood glucose is moving in and how quickly it is changing. It also provides some suggestions of what action could be taken by the pump user to maintain glycaemic stability. The intermittent use of sensors for three-day periods can provide pump users with a large amount of information that can be analysed to identify trends in blood glucose levels and insulin requirements, and help them to programme their infusion rates to more closely match their needs. NHS funding for this type of monitoring system is limited, although pump users can choose to fund their own continuous glucose monitoring sensors if they wish.

## Calculation of bolus doses

Some insulin pumps can provide suggestions of what bolus doses should be taken. To use this function, the pump user programmes in their target blood glucose range and the insulin ratios they are using to match their carbohydrate intake and/or to correct high blood glucose readings. If food is eaten, the pump user then programmes in the amount of carbohydrate this contains, and the pump provides a suggestion of how much insulin to give as a bolus. If the blood glucose level is too high, again this can be programmed into the pump (or with some pumps will already be in the pump) and a suggested correction dose will be provided. Some pumps can also take account of bolus doses that have recently been given, to avoid a new bolus overlapping with previous boluses and causing too much insulin to be given within a short space of time. In all cases, the pump user still has the choice of whether to give the suggested amount of insulin, rather than the pump automatically delivering the suggested bolus dose. This means that pump users can account for their personal circumstances, for example, if they are about to undertake physical activity, they might wish to give a reduced bolus dose.

The pumps available in the United Kingdom vary regarding the type of bolus calculations they offer, and individual pump manufacturers will be able to provide more information on their specific models. It is likely that this type of function will be incorporated into most newer models of pumps as they are produced, and also this type of function is likely to increase in sophistication as technology advances.

## Computer download facility

Most of the pumps have optional computer software that might either be accessed via a website, be provided with the pump or need to be purchased separately. If the pump memory is downloaded into a computer, the pump user can see a much larger picture of insulin doses and trends, and also store these results for longer-term analysis. Some programs provide insulin pump data only, some provide blood glucose meter readings only and some provide both, which can be viewed together on one chart. These charts might be able to be emailed to health professionals or be directly accessed via an Internet link so that results can be discussed either electronically or by phone, reducing the need to attend appointments. In some cases, the information can automatically be made available to both the pump user and the health professional. Some pump users find this facility extremely helpful, but it does require more work on their part (see Chapter Three for their reflections on how useful they find this).

## Customising some of the pump functions

Some insulin pumps can be customised to suit the individual pump user, although the features that can be customised will vary from one pump to another. In some, the pump user can choose to use a menu with all the available programs or simplify their menu to hold the basic functions only. Alarms can be customised in some, for example they can be set to remind the pump user to check their blood glucose a set period after a bolus has been given. Another example is that the pump user can set time frames for the alarms to remind them if they have missed a food bolus or if they need to change their infusion set.

Other aspects which can be customised include the maximum bolus dose that can be given, which provides a safety net if someone is concerned about accidentally programming too high an amount. Being able to customise a pump can be helpful if someone is concerned they might forget to carry out some pump functions, and can also help the pump user by reducing the number of steps they need to take to use the different programs on the pump.

## Programmable via a computer

Some pumps can be programmed using a computer, rather than the infusion rates being programmed directly into the pump, and the computer-generated information is downloaded into the pump ready for use. The main advantage of this is that the pump user can see more information at the same time on a computer screen, rather than looking at individual settings on the pump.

## Ability to set low hourly basal rates

The pumps vary regarding how small a dose they can deliver per hour, from 0.1 units per hour to 0.025 units per hour. The lower rates can be useful for children and babies requiring extremely small insulin doses, and can mean that the need to dilute insulin for these small doses is avoided.

## Storage of food carbohydrate values

Some of the pumps allow the user to store information about a number of different types of food, together with their carbohydrate value. This can save pump users from carrying around carbohydrate reference guides, and also allows them to keep records of the carbohydrate content of many of the foods they commonly eat so that they can quickly access the information rather than have to recalculate each time.

## Creating meal boluses for future use

This function allows pump users to create a number of specific meal boluses to use, which helps if they are regularly eating food of similar carbohydrate value and type, as they can recall the specific bolus instead of reprogramming a new amount. Programming in a food bolus for a packed lunch that might vary very little from one day to the next is one example of when this might be useful.

## Remote control

A remote control is available for some pumps, which can be used to programme bolus doses without having to physically handle the pump. This can be convenient in social situations and also for managing pumps in young children, particularly when used in combination with the keylock feature.

## Using a prefilled insulin cartridge

One of the models of available pumps is designed to hold a 3 ml (millilitres) prefilled insulin cartridge, giving the advantage of not having to draw insulin up into a small reservoir before inserting it into the pump. While this is more convenient, it also means that the pump is slightly larger to accommodate the cartridge and the plunger, and only the specific insulin cartridge made by one company is recommended, to ensure the accuracy of small doses of insulin being delivered.

## Variable insulin reservoir size

The amount of insulin that a pump will hold varies from one model to another, and also, with some models, the pump user can choose what size insulin reservoir to use. If a pump user needs larger doses of insulin, the larger reservoir will help reduce the number of times they need to change the reservoir.

## Integrated blood glucose meter

Integrating blood glucose measuring with an insulin pump is a key aim of many of the pump manufacturers. Using the continuous monitor as described earlier in this section is one option; another is for a meter that remains separate but can be attached to the back of the pump, which means that the pump user does not have to carry their meter around. The use of this type of device is limited and is not available in all parts of the world.

## Memory of previously programmed settings

Some pumps retain information in their memory regarding the previous settings that have been used, for example the amount by which a temporary basal rate has been increased or decreased, together with how long it was programmed for, can be saved. The next time the pump user accesses that function, they have the option of activating the retained information or of programming a new setting, depending on their needs at the time.

## Rotating the display

One of the pumps has the option of rotating the display by 180 degrees so that, whichever way up someone chooses to wear their pump, they can see the display clearly. This feature is particularly useful for left-handed pump users.

## Availability of loan pumps

Some manufacturers offer pump users the option of borrowing a spare insulin pump to take on holiday with them, if travelling abroad. This can give people peace of mind, although taking supplies in case of needing to revert back to injection therapy is always still recommended (this is discussed more fully in Chapter 12).

## INFUSION SETS

With all pumps, there is a variety of infusion sets to choose from, in terms of type of needle or cannula and also the length of the tubing to attach the pump to its user. Some infusion sets are produced by the pump manufacturers and are recommended for use specifically for the companies' own insulin pumps. Other infusion sets are produced by independent companies. For those pump companies that do not produce their own infusion sets, any standard infusion set with a luer lock connection can be used.

Most needles and cannulae come in a range of sizes, with the option of using different lengths of tubing, and some also have automatic insertion devices. The features of individual types of infusion sets are discussed below, although it is important to recognise that there is no single infusion set that is superior in safety or effectiveness than any other, and the choice of type of infusion set should be based on the pump user's preference unless clinical needs dictate otherwise.

Some people might experience initial discomfort when first inserting a new needle or cannula, but this should disappear within two hours of insertion, whichever type of infusion set is used. If the infusion site continues feeling uncomfortable, the needle or cannula might need to be removed and a new one inserted. If a pump user has ongoing difficulties, a variety of infusion sets should be tried until the most comfortable and effective one is identified. This section outlines the features of different infusion sets and their practical use.

## Choosing a needle or cannula

A stainless steel needle, which should be replaced every two days, or a Teflon cannula, which should be replaced every three days, are the two types of devices that can be used to infuse the insulin subcutaneously. Stainless steel needles, which are inserted at a 90-degree angle, are arguably the most simple to insert. Cannulae can be slightly more complex: some of them are designed to be inserted at around a 45-degree angle to the skin; others, at 90 degrees. It is important to refer to the individual manufacturer's guidelines on how to insert a specific cannula or needle. A cannula might need slightly firmer pressure to puncture the skin, and care needs to be taken that the needle doesn't dislodge from the cannula prior to insertion. Some pump users choose needles for their simplicity; others, particularly those who are concerned about the safety and comfort of having a needle that remains in their skin 24 hours a day, prefer to use a cannula with a removable needle.

## Length of needle or cannula

The needle lengths for infusion sets inserted at a 90-degree angle to the skin vary from six to 12 millimetres, and for some inserted at an angle the length can be up to 17 millimetres to achieve the same depth in the subcutaneous tissue. While people might opt for the shortest needle or cannula, some prefer a slightly longer one as they feel it is less likely to dislodge. The assessment of cannula or needle length can be helped by how comfortable it feels: if it does not reach an adequate depth in the subcutaneous tissue, the pump user can experience a stinging sensation every time they give a bolus; if it is too deep, it is likely to feel uncomfortable most of the time. Using these parameters as general guidance can help to determine the right needle length for an individual. If someone has very little subcutaneous fat, a hydrocolloid dressing might need to be put on the skin and the needle inserted through this to ensure it does not penetrate too deeply.

# Length of tubing

As with the infusion set options, individual preferences play an important part in deciding what length of tubing to use. They vary from 30 to 110 centimetres long, although different manufacturers will each produce a range of between two and four lengths to choose from. Short tubing lengths mean there is less tubing to be tucked away into pockets or under belts, so can reduce the chances of catching the tubing on door handles and other objects. Longer tubing can help the pump user handle the pump easily without pulling on the infusion site. Most people will develop a preference for a tubing length but might also choose to vary this in specific circumstances, for example they might need longer tubing if their pump is strapped to their thigh than if it is worn on their belt.

## Insertion devices

Some of the infusion sets have an automatic insertion device to put the needle into the skin; others are inserted manually. Some insertion devices also retract the removed needle so that it can be disposed of safely. Again, the personal preference of the pump user should play a part in whether this influences the type of infusion set chosen.

## CONCLUSION

This chapter has provided an overview of the features of insulin pumps, both general and specific, and of infusion sets in common use in the United Kingdom. Technology is advancing at a rapid pace, and it is likely that many more companies will be providing insulin pumps in the near future and also that the insulin pump features will become increasingly sophisticated, to be able to deliver insulin in a more physiological way. Pumps that suggest insulin doses based on parameters and targets set by the individual pump user are likely to become more commonly used, reducing the need for complicated calculations on the part of the pump user. It is important to remember that it is not just the technology that is important but also the support and after-sales service provided by the manufacturing companies, much of which determines whether pump users feel confident and helps them to increase their success in managing their diabetes with their chosen pump.

Chapter 5
# Setting up an Insulin Pump Service

When first starting to use insulin pumps in a diabetes team, planning ahead regarding the organisation of the service and how it might develop in the future is one of the key steps to take. This ensures that using pump therapy doesn't place additional stress on existing services and commitments, it allows time to plan ahead regarding funding, it helps to identify what training is required and for whom and, most importantly, it ensures that people with diabetes who are starting to use pumps can access appropriate help and support. It also helps avoid an insulin pump service running into difficulties in the future, either through a lack of staffing or funding or through competing with other diabetes service priorities. This chapter will look at the different organisational aspects that should be considered when developing an insulin pump service.

## PRE-PLANNING

Involving the whole of the diabetes team in developing a philosophy and planning how the service is to be organised are the first steps to ensuring the success of an insulin pump service. The greater the consensus between team members, the less chance there is for any misunderstanding of roles, different messages being passed around or for resentment to build between team members. People with diabetes should also be involved as early as possible – Section 11 of the Health and Social Care Act (Department of Health, 2001) outlines that service users should be involved at every stage of service planning, delivery and evaluation, and user involvement in pump services is supported by the Insulin Pumps Working Group (Department of Health, 2007). Even in areas where insulin pumps have not yet been used, many people with diabetes will still be able to identify what is important for them in relation to service provision, and should be included in discussions.

The key areas that should be looked at when planning an insulin pump service, which will be discussed in turn, are:

- developing an insulin pump service philosophy
- level of service provision
- selection criteria to assess suitability for using a pump
- funding pathways
- organisation and structure of the service
- who will be involved: roles and responsibilities
- access to courses for health professionals
- which pumps to use
- educational literature for pump users
- literature for health professionals
- record-keeping for pump users
- measuring the success of an insulin pump service.

When an insulin pump service is being planned in advance, as already stated, involving all team members in creating a vision of the service will increase everyone's understanding and their commitment to its development, particularly for those who might not be as directly involved. It can be easy for one or two enthusiastic team members to try and develop the service in isolation from other team members, but this is likely to produce a less stable service in the long term, for example, if one of the enthusiastic members left the team, the remaining one might find it difficult to continue without the support of others. Support from the whole team is therefore essential, but it is still likely that there will only be a small number of key people who will be more involved and who will play a major part in providing the service. Recognising that it takes enthusiasts to move a service forward, but also recognising that a pump service is not everyone's priority, will help to get the balance between resources committed to an insulin pump service and those committed to other service developments.

## DEVELOPING AN INSULIN PUMP SERVICE PHILOSOPHY

Agreeing in advance what the team's core beliefs are, and what approach to insulin pump therapy will be taken, provides a sound basis for building a service, as well as helping the team work more closely together. It will also reduce interprofessional variation and increase equity of service provision.

The first step is to explore what each team member believes about insulin pumps, and a variety of questions and discussions can be used to achieve

**Table 5.1**   Questions for use in developing a team philosophy

Do you believe insulin pumps are beneficial or a positive therapy option to use?
If you had diabetes, would you want to use a pump?
What drawbacks do you see in using insulin pumps?
What are your biggest concerns about using insulin pumps?
How would you rate your confidence in the safety of insulin pumps?

this. Examples of questions that can be helpful for individuals to consider are listed in Table 5.1. Working through these or similar questions will enable all team members to express their views and to explore what they believe are the pros and cons of using insulin pumps and will ensure that people's beliefs and concerns are based on reality rather than assumptions. Following these discussions, it will be possible to work together to decide on a team philosophy, often expressed in a number of statements, for example: 'anyone expressing an interest in using insulin pump therapy should have the opportunity to discuss it further' or 'any person considered suitable for using insulin pump therapy will be discussed at a team meeting'.

The most important aspect of any philosophy is that all team members subscribe to it. To do this, they should all have the opportunity to contribute their ideas, and they should all be reasonably comfortable with the outcome. If different team members hold extremely opposing views, this will take time and effort to achieve, and the resulting philosophy is likely to be a compromise between the different views. However, particularly for those who are less enthusiastic, the philosophy can provide reassurance that the insulin pump service is not going to be developed solely on the basis of the opinions of a few team members only and also that it won't result in sacrificing other equally important aspects of the diabetes service.

## LEVEL OF SERVICE PROVISION

Identifying how much involvement the diabetes team would like to have with insulin pump therapy will help with service planning. There are a number of service models that have been developed within the United Kingdom, as described in the remainder of this section.

## Referral to a neighbouring specialist diabetes team

In some areas, where either it is anticipated that the numbers of people requiring insulin pumps will be small or a centre of excellence is close by, the decision might be made to not initiate pump therapy in that service but to refer to the neighbouring specialist diabetes team. If this is the case, the amount of ongoing care that is required from the referring team depends on how much is provided by the centre of excellence.

One option is for the centre of excellence to provide care for an individual during the assessment and early days on a pump and then to refer back to the original diabetes service for the provision of ongoing care. This means that expertise within the referring service will need to be developed to take on this role, to be able to provide support and ongoing care in pump therapy. National guidance suggests that specialist teams initiating insulin pump therapy also have the responsibility of ensuring they are referring back to a team which is competent and confident to provide ongoing care (Department of Health, 2007).

An alternative model would be for the centre of excellence to provide not only the initial care and training but also regular reviews as part of their care package. If this is the case, the amount of input the referring team is likely to have into pump management will be extremely limited, although annual reviews and other aspects of care might still need to be provided, including emergency care.

Referral to a centre of excellence reduces the need for a large amount of specialist knowledge to be developed by the original diabetes team, although some expertise will still be needed. In areas that are highly populated, such as large cities, this model might make economic sense, but in rural areas, and as insulin pump therapy becomes more widely used, it is likely that the development of local expertise will become necessary in the long term.

## Providing a service with support from pump manufacturers

This type of service means that most of the care is provided from within the diabetes team and that the pump manufacturers might provide some aspects of care. For example, a trainer external to the diabetes team might initiate pump therapy and provide the initial care required, with the diabetes team then providing ongoing care. One advantage of this model is that the assessment of the individual prior to the initiation of pump therapy, and the initial training, will be provided by trainers with a wide experience in this field. It also means that one of the more time-consuming aspects of pump therapy can be provided with minimal impact on the diabetes service and the time of the health professionals available. In many areas, honorary contracts will be required for any external trainers providing this type of service.

There are some drawbacks to this option. First, the training is usually provided by people employed by the pump manufacturer and is based on an agreement to use a pump manufactured by that company. Arguably, some bias might be introduced into the assessment, and pump therapy might be initiated slightly more readily than if the assessment were carried out by the diabetes team. Also, the trainer has no prior knowledge of, or contact with, the pump user, whereas members of the diabetes team might know the individual well. If external pump trainers are used regularly, anecdotally the diabetes team are likely to build up their own expertise much more slowly than if they were providing their own insulin pump training. The pump manufacturers historically provided this service as a way of diabetes teams learning how to manage insulin pump therapy, and if used in this way it can be extremely beneficial to be initiating pump therapy in partnership, as it will help diabetes team members gain the necessary skills to manage pump therapy in the future. If the pump training is being carried out without any diabetes team members present, however, the diabetes team are unlikely to develop their own skills, which might promote a longer-term reliance on the pump manufacturer. There might also be some legal considerations, particularly if the external trainer is involved in determining the starting doses of insulin.

## Providing a complete insulin pump service

If a specialist diabetes team decides to provide a complete service for pump users in the area, including pre-pump assessment, pump initiation and ongoing care, the service needs to be structured to enable this to happen. See the section 'Organisation and structure of the service' for more information on how to do this.

## Providing a tertiary referral service for other areas

A fourth option is to provide not only a complete service for pump users locally but also a tertiary referral service to which other diabetes teams can refer. Most specialist diabetes teams that currently accept tertiary referrals developed their expertise at a time when pump therapy was being used in very small numbers of people in the United Kingdom, so the service might have provided for a wide geographical area. However, with many areas looking at cost-effective models of care, this model might be chosen to be developed from the outset, with agreement between the local diabetes teams that they will refer potential pump users to the service.

If this option is chosen, additional aspects will need to be considered. Calculating the number of people with diabetes that might be referred, based on the size of the population serviced by the referring diabetes teams, will help determine the resources required. The costing of the service is important, to ensure that financial arrangements closely match the actual costs of the service. Also, referral systems, the amount of care to be provided and communication systems should be determined.

## SELECTION CRITERIA TO ASSESS SUITABILITY FOR USING A PUMP

NICE guidance, outlined in Chapter One, remains relatively narrow regarding the types of people for whom insulin pump therapy is recommended. In reality, there are likely to be many more people who would benefit from using a pump than a strict interpretation of the guidance would suggest, and Chapter Six discusses selection criteria that might be used. In order to be able to provide insulin pumps for those who would benefit, it is important to agree as a team what the local selection criteria are going to be. In those diabetes specialist teams that have developed their own criteria, a broader interpretation of NICE guidance is often used, for example they might include people whose lifestyle is the main reason for considering pump therapy.

Once local criteria have been developed, these should be revisited at regular intervals, as the specialist pump team will develop greater expertise and are likely to identify a wider group of people who might benefit from using an insulin pump.

There are also people in specialist categories not covered by NICE guidance but who find it extremely difficult to manage their diabetes using other forms of insulin delivery. These include people with insulin allergies or with an extreme sensitivity to even small doses of insulin. It is difficult to categorise which individual circumstances will indicate a clinical need for using an insulin pump, so cases such as these are likely to need consideration on an individual basis.

## FUNDING PATHWAYS

Since the introduction of NICE guidance in 2003 in relation to pump therapy, the NHS has more readily provided funding for the use of insulin pumps, whereas prior to the guidance being published many people with diabetes had to fund their own pumps and the ongoing costs of consumables. It is mandatory for primary care organisations (PCOs) to implement NICE guidance, but there will be variation in how the guidance on insulin pumps is interpreted, as described above. PCOs and diabetes teams need to develop local agreements on what selection criteria will be adopted for pump use, based on the guidance but also allowing for the consideration of individual cases, as already discussed, to ensure that insulin pumps are available to those who will benefit from using the therapy.

PCOs might be keen to set specific budgets in relation to insulin pump therapy, to help their financial planning process. Carrying out a local population needs assessment is recommended, as this can help to assess how many people are likely to benefit from using insulin pump therapy, which in turn will facilitate realistic budget-setting. In some areas, PCOs and diabetes teams agree a specific number of new pump users per year whose treatment will be funded, as well as supporting ongoing pump users. With this system, waiting lists are developed to keep within budgets and regular reviews are undertaken to negotiate gradual increases in the annual numbers of new pump users, although it could be argued that this is restricting access to insulin pumps for some who might benefit from using them. In other areas, PCOs will fund anyone who fits the local, or NICE, criteria. Whichever system is adopted, it is important for diabetes teams to see enough people to gain expertise in this clinical area. There is no minimum number of people using insulin pumps that a service should care for, but it is recommended that services with small numbers of pump users should develop strong links with a bigger service (Department of Health, 2007).

## Accessing funding

Once funding is agreed, a system needs to be put in place to allow access to the funding. An option used in some areas of the United Kingdom is for the diabetes team to apply to the PCO for funding for each individual who has been identified as suitable for using an insulin pump and to gain approval each time before initiating the therapy. In other areas, the diabetes team have the freedom to initiate insulin pump therapy in those people who are considered suitable (still in accordance with local criteria), and then the PCO is notified after the event. As insulin pump therapy becomes a more normal part of providing a specialist diabetes service, and possibly if insulin pumps become cheaper through technological advances and more widespread use, these issues should be resolved and funding might become available on a less restrictive basis.

## ORGANISATION AND STRUCTURE OF THE SERVICE

Even with careful planning, it can be difficult to develop the perfect system, as service needs might change with greater numbers of people starting to use insulin pump therapy. As discussed earlier, as the insulin pump team gain expertise, it is likely that more people with diabetes will be identified as potentially benefiting from pump therapy than had originally been anticipated. The initial organisation of the service should identify the immediate needs but might also include plans for expansion as the demand for the service increases. A new insulin pump service will need to include: how people will be assessed prior to using an insulin pump, whether separate clinics will be set up, how initial education and training will be provided, what ongoing support and follow-up will be offered and what emergency care will be available.

## Pre-pump assessment

Chapter Six discusses the complexity of assessing an individual's suitability for using an insulin pump. To ensure that those who might benefit from using insulin pumps can gain access to them, any assessment process should include a structure for identifying who might initially be considered and what form the assessment will take from then on, possibly through the development of an insulin pump pathway. As well as providing a framework for health professionals, this will also mean that people with diabetes will have a clear understanding of the likelihood of them needing, or being able to access, pump therapy.

There are a number of service models that could be adopted:

- Anyone expressing an interest in an insulin pump is referred to one health professional, who provides information and carries out all the initial assessments regarding the suitability of using a pump, using criteria agreed by the whole diabetes team. In this model, it is often the diabetes specialist nurse who carries out the assessment, although there is likely to be consultation with others before the final decision is made. This method means that the assessment process is likely to be more equitable as it is carried out by one person, but it also means that the rest of the diabetes team build up less expertise as they are not involved in the assessment process.
- Pre-pump assessments are carried out jointly between two health professionals. In this scenario, the two people involved would be likely to be a diabetes specialist nurse and a consultant diabetologist. This ensures that personal bias does not influence the decisions, and so potentially a more objective view is gained. And also, discussion of each person's situation might help the decision-making process. As in the first option, it might exclude the rest of the diabetes team to a great extent.

- All the diabetes team develop skills in carrying out a basic assessment for insulin pump therapy, and people will only be referred for more in-depth assessment if they fit the team's criteria. This model requires the whole of the diabetes team to gain some skills in insulin pump therapy, to be able to provide initial information and to understand who might benefit from using a pump, but it still allows for further assessment by the team members specialising in pump therapy.

Discussing the above or other options within the diabetes team will contribute to how the service will be organised, including finding time to carry out the pre-pump assessments, either within the routine appointment and review system or with additional time being set aside.

## Separate insulin pump clinics

In some areas, specialist insulin pump clinics are set up, in much the same way that other specialist clinics, such as pregnancy, are organised. Separate clinics provide the advantages of all the specialist team members being available and being able to communicate easily with each other to ensure a smooth continuity of care. It can also help the health professionals involved to focus specifically on pumps during that time and means that appropriate timings for assessment and review appointments can be allocated. The alternative is to see pump users and potential pump users in the same clinics as everyone else, which might be preferred as it normalises pump use as simply an alternative treatment.

For diabetes teams just starting to use insulin pumps, if a separate clinic is set up, it could be run fairly infrequently, for example once a month, until the numbers of people attending grow. Or the initial small number of people could be seen within the existing service, while plans to expand the service as demand grows could be put in place.

Whichever method is decided upon, it is important that the time allocated for appointments permits adequate discussion and assessment. Also, when initiating pump therapy, it might be necessary to devote the equivalent of one or two whole days to initiating pump therapy for one person, although this can be divided into a number of manageable time periods (see Chapter Nine for more information on initiating pump therapy). It is likely, for health professionals just beginning to use pumps, that longer appointments will initially be needed, as with learning anything new. This will allow time for health professionals to gain confidence in using the pumps, carrying out assessments and providing information to pump users, all of which will become easier with experience.

## Initial education and training for pump users

Education and training for people starting to use an insulin pump can be time-consuming, however it is provided. Group education is becoming the norm in many aspects of diabetes care where people are learning new skills in managing their diabetes, and initiating pump therapy is ideal for this. People with diabetes also report that they find interaction with other pump users, particularly in the initial stages, to be extremely helpful (see Chapter Three for more information). How to approach educating people about using an insulin pump is discussed in Chapter Eight, and developing a comprehensive training plan is discussed in Chapter Nine. Planning how the education of pump users is to be integrated into a diabetes service, particularly when they are first starting to use a pump, will help to ensure that adequate time and expertise is allocated to this.

## Ongoing support and follow-up

Planning clinic structures should include not only time for pre-pump assessments and initiation of insulin pump therapy but also consideration for what type of follow-up system will be developed. In the initial weeks or months of someone using an insulin pump for the first time, they are likely to need a high level of support, possibly with frequent contact either through face-to-face appointments, by telephone or email. Some pump users describe the experience as similar to when they were first diagnosed, as they are learning a very different way of managing their diabetes. Because of this, it can be an opportunity for them to revisit many aspects of their diabetes care (for example how to manage physical activity, drinking alcohol or eating out), and up-to-date information and a significant amount of input from health professionals at this time can be of real benefit in helping people develop coping strategies and problem-solving skills for the future. Chapter Nine provides more information about follow-up in the early days of pump therapy.

Anecdotally, after three to six months of using an insulin pump, people develop confidence in managing the therapy, and are likely to need much less frequent contact with health professionals. They also might be less receptive to new information and ideas on how to manage their diabetes using an insulin pump, as they will have developed their own ways of managing the therapy in situations they commonly encounter, and as a result might be more easily able to apply what they have learnt to new situations. There will always be people who are exceptions to this, for example people who have learning difficulties, gastroparesis or other complicated physical needs might require a high level of ongoing support, so a system which allows some people to have close contact in the longer term should also exist.

So, to deliver an effective insulin pump service, recognition within the diabetes team of the need for increased contact in the early stages of therapy is important, and working together to identify how this can be achieved will again help the pump service become an integrated part of a diabetes service. For longer-term follow-up, routine medical reviews will be required as for non-pump users, but more frequent appointments with a diabetes specialist nurse and/or dietitian will be helpful for many, to discuss the aspects of managing diabetes specifically in relation to pump therapy.

## Access to emergency care

Accessibility to help and support in an emergency should be considered, and service models vary between specialist teams in this respect. Some diabetes services have a team member on call, possibly on a rotational basis. While, anecdotally, they are rarely contacted, were this system to be implemented, its organisational and financial implications need to be considered. It could be argued that, if 24-hour access were required for pump users, this should be available for all people with diabetes, regardless of whether they use insulin pumps or not. In reality, 24-hour cover within the NHS is provided via primary care services and accident and emergency departments, neither of which are likely to have a great deal of in-depth experience of insulin pump therapy. It therefore follows that access to specialist help is unlikely to be available outside normal working hours, so a diabetes service might have to clarify what people should do in an emergency, for example if they damage their pump or suspect it of malfunctioning. A common-sense approach, adopted by many insulin pump services, is to provide pump users with information on how to revert back to injection therapy as a short-term emergency measure until they are able to access more specialist advice, either from the diabetes team or from the pump manufacturer. Specific emergency situations, for example suspected ketoacidosis, should also be highlighted as requiring emergency care, rather than as something that pump users can manage for themselves. It is important to clarify the emergency care aspect of service organisation and how it will work in practice.

## WHO WILL BE INVOLVED: ROLES AND RESPONSIBILITIES

In many insulin pump services in the United Kingdom, it is common for diabetes teams to have one consultant, one diabetes specialist nurse and one dietitian as the core members of the insulin pump team, which equates to the national recommendations for a specialist insulin pump team (National Institute for Health and Clinical Excellence, 2003). In other areas, a team philosophy of everyone gaining expertise has been developed, particularly in areas where different team members cover a widespread geographical area. When first starting out, it might be prudent for a small number of team members to gain insulin pump experience and expertise before involving the wider diabetes team. If taking this approach, a long-term plan of how people are going to access training and become involved over time can ensure realistic service planning for the future.

Once it has been identified who is to be involved, it is useful to decide what part each health professional will play in providing the service. This involves developing a clear assessment process, including which health professionals will see people at different stages, as well as who will provide different aspects of insulin pump education. Diabetes teams experienced in pump therapy report that as their expertise has developed they often find that some aspects of their roles become interchangeable. This could mean that a specialist dietitian might have input into insulin dose adjustment or that a specialist nurse might take on more of a role in pre-pump assessment. In most diabetes teams, the diabetes specialist nurse devotes the greatest time to insulin pump therapy, but this might not always be the case.

The more clearly team members' roles are defined, the easier it will be to set up the service and also to identify the training requirements for each person, as discussed in the next section. It is also important, however, to ensure there is good communication between team members and easy ways to gain access to each other, particularly in the early days of using insulin pumps, when most team members will be relative novices in this field. It is useful to build in regular opportunities to review cases and share ideas and experiences, possibly at diabetes team meetings, which will help the overall expertise of team members to develop as well as reduce the likelihood of people with diabetes receiving conflicting messages.

There might be a number of people within the diabetes team who do not become involved in the specialist service. These team members are likely to see people with diabetes who might benefit from pump therapy but who are unlikely to come into contact with the core insulin pump team as part of their usual care, so the team need to decide how pumps are to be discussed in these situations. Care needs to be taken to ensure that people are not unfairly judged as unsuitable simply because the health professional they are seeing has limited insulin pump knowledge or has specific beliefs about the use of insulin pumps, although developing a team philosophy as described earlier in this chapter can help reduce the potential for this.

Developing a care pathway is one way of increasing the likelihood of people being treated equitably and receiving similar information about insulin pumps, as discussed later in this chapter. Posters in waiting areas can help people attending clinics to be more aware of the insulin pump service and who it might be suitable for, and other sources of information, such as a list of websites, could be provided.

## Psychological input into the service

Psychological input into an insulin pump service is a useful addition. In some areas, a psychologist is involved as part of the routine assessment of potential pump users; in other areas, criteria have been developed to help identify when referral to a psychologist should be considered. As well as determining what role a psychologist could play in the service, it can also be useful to consider what psychological training is required for members of the diabetes team.

Training can help health professionals identify earlier when psychological issues are causing difficulties, which results in people with diabetes getting the help and support they need, either within the consultation or through onward referral. For some, simply wearing a pump has a huge psychological impact, but there might also be psychological aspects that could indicate which people might get more benefit from using a pump and which people might benefit less, as discussed in Chapter Six.

## ACCESS TO COURSES FOR HEALTH PROFESSIONALS

Identifying the training and education requirements of the core insulin pump team, and of the wider diabetes team, is crucial to the success of a service. There are a number of courses available, most of which were developed by the diabetes teams in the United Kingdom who were involved in the research trials into pump therapy in the 1980s. There is no single course that is seen as the gold standard, and NICE guidance simply states that pump therapy 'should be initiated only by a trained specialist team' (National Institute for Health and Clinical Excellence, 2003) but does not specify what that training should be. Considering the team's needs should be the first priority when deciding what course to access.

## Accreditation of courses

Some insulin pump courses do not hold academic accreditation but provide a great deal of expertise in the practical aspects of using insulin pumps in clinical practice. Accredited short courses are also available, most at master's degree level, set up either by universities or by diabetes teams with clinical expertise, and students attending these usually have the choice of whether to undertake the accreditation route or simply attend the course. Some of the insulin pump manufacturers also run courses, and there are also courses provided by independent insulin pump trainers that can be run for local diabetes teams.

## Specific considerations when choosing a course

If specific expertise is required, for example if insulin pumps will be used in pregnancy or paediatrics, it is important to access a course that includes coverage of those aspects. Other factors that might influence the choice of course could be the locality of the course, availability of places, recommendations from other diabetes teams and which insulin pumps are preferred by the diabetes team. It can be beneficial for a number of health professionals from the same diabetes team to attend a course together, particularly if the service is in its infancy.

The length of courses varies, generally from two to four days, and, while the shorter courses should not necessarily be chosen simply because they take less time from the working week, that might be an influencing factor. Cost might also be a consideration, particularly with the cost of academically accredited modules being driven by university standards, which has introduced large variations. In some cases, pump manufacturers actively support courses and sponsor health professionals to attend, as this helps diabetes teams new to insulin pump therapy to get started. Pump manufacturers might also run their own courses, either for a wide geographical area or locally for a diabetes team.

## Course content

Most insulin pump training courses will offer the opportunity for participants to wear an insulin pump containing saline for at least 24 hours. Setting up the pump, programming basal rates, calculating and giving bolus doses in relation to carbohydrate intake and wearing the pump overnight all help participants to familiarise themselves with the experiences of pump users, as well as providing an introduction to the day-to-day decision-making required for successful pump use. On some courses, everyone wears the same pump; on others, there might be a choice of which pump to use, or there might be an opportunity to handle and wear a number of different pumps during the course. In all cases, wearing the pump for a few days is unlikely to result in the details of using the pumps being remembered, but it does provide a starting point, and the pump manufacturers will provide ample opportunities for becoming more familiar with the models chosen for use by the diabetes team.

## Gaining experience in the early days

Having completed a course, the next step is to gain experience in insulin pump therapy. One option is to start using insulin pumps in the diabetes service, with support from the pump manufacturers. Another is to develop close relationships with a diabetes team who have already set up their insulin pump service, possibly to visit their clinics and see how pump therapy is managed in reality, and gain experience in this way. A third option is to be mentored by an existing pump service, whereby their experience and expertise can be used alongside developing the new service. Whatever the preferred method, having some form of back-up and access to people who can answer questions as they arise, and provide support in whatever form is needed, will result in expertise being developed much more quickly than working in isolation.

## WHICH PUMPS TO USE

Deciding which pumps to use in a diabetes service is difficult with limited experience, and decisions at this stage are likely to be fairly arbitrary. An ideal service would offer people the choice of all available insulin pumps, but, for diabetes teams new to pump therapy, becoming familiar with one or two pumps initially would be prudent, in order to be able to confidently and competently help pump users accessing the service. Over time, the pump choice might be broadened as confidence is gained.

Pump manufacturers will provide information about and demonstrations of their pumps, and will also outline the type of support and other services they can provide. There are a number of different criteria to determine what pumps to use in what area. These can include:

- support from the pump manufacturers
- features of the individual pumps
- pump users' preferences.

## Support from the pump manufacturers

The pump manufacturers provide support in many different ways, which can be a key factor in deciding which pumps to use. The types of support that can be offered are: training courses for health professionals, easy access for ongoing support, demonstration pumps and educational literature. The service they provide for pump users is also important, possibly even more so, as they need to have adequate back-up services if the pumps malfunction and have easy access if pump users have queries they need answering. If a company provides very poor support services, this will reflect on the service provided by the diabetes team and can make it extremely difficult to run an efficient and effective insulin pump service. As pump therapy grows, newer companies are likely to be developing products, and identifying what support is available from the company should be one of the criteria to help decide whether to use those pumps.

## Features of individual pumps

Pump features might be one of the criteria to use when choosing an insulin pump. Pumps produced by different companies often have many different features, for example how they deliver their insulin boluses, what their dose range and variability of programming the basal rate is, what size of insulin reservoir they have or whether they use prefilled cartridges, what choice of bolus options there are, whether they can be operated by remote control and how easy the button-pressing sequences are to use. (More information on the pump features available can be found in Chapter Four.) If pump features are used as one of the main criteria, it is important to avoid personal bias or preference being the overriding factor, as the features preferred by a health professional might not be those that individual pump users feel are important to them.

## Pump users' preferences

It is important to take pump users' preferences into account. While 'patient choice' is repeatedly stated by the Government as something to be strived for, in reality choice is often limited by health professionals and budget-holders in view of some of the constraints and considerations discussed above. If people are given complete choice to decide which pump to use, they should also have access to information and demonstrations of all the pumps. However this is approached, it can be a time-consuming exercise, and it might be worth adopting a pragmatic approach by using a small number of pumps within a service initially until more confidence is gained, but also allowing people with diabetes who wish to explore using other pumps to carry out their own research, for example via the Internet, to make an informed choice of which pump is right for them.

## EDUCATIONAL LITERATURE FOR PUMP USERS

Written literature is important, initially to help people learn about pump therapy and decide whether it is the right option for them, as well as providing information about dealing with the technical aspects and day-to-day issues of insulin pumps, such as undertaking physical activity, eating out or managing hyperglycaemia. NICE guidance (2003) highlights that a diabetes team should agree a 'common core of advice' for pump users, which includes the messages contained in educational literature.

There is an abundance of educational leaflets and literature available from the pump manufacturers, and it is important to identify which of these are the most useful. Many of the introductory leaflets are fairly generic in the way they explain the benefits of insulin pumps and can be useful, when the idea of pump therapy is first discussed, for people with diabetes to take away, read and show to others close to them.

The companies also produce written information specific to their pumps, which is important as it will take pump users through the different pump features and how to use them, and will usually also include a trouble-shooting guide if the pump user is having difficulty with a particular aspect of the pump. Most of this literature is provided for use at the time when pump therapy is initiated and might include small, portable, quick-reference guides.

Lifestyle and day-to-day advice leaflets, while also available from the pump manufacturers, might or might not match the information the diabetes team feel is important, so looking at each leaflet individually will help the team decide which is appropriate to use.

Another option is to produce literature unique to the diabetes team. While this has the disadvantage of needing additional time and effort, it can allow the team to encompass the local organisation of a service, such as when clinics are held, who the specialist pump team are, where to get pump supplies from and what action is recommended in varying circumstances. It also means that the diabetes team can ensure that the specific messages they feel important are included, for example how insulin doses can be assessed and adjusted. For diabetes teams starting out with insulin pump therapy, it might be helpful to use the pump manufacturers' literature initially and to develop local literature as the need arises.

## LITERATURE FOR HEALTH PROFESSIONALS

It is also important to identify what policies and protocols will be needed locally. For example, there might be many situations where non-pump specialists will be interacting with pump users, and producing guidance for different situations can help. Accident and emergency departments are likely to need some basic guidelines that explain how insulin pump therapy works, to prevent them detaching an insulin pump from an unconscious person without substituting a different method of insulin delivery. Similarly, ambulance services might require some written information. It can also be useful to provide general practitioners with specific information when someone registered at their surgery starts to use a pump, to help them be able to have useful conversations with the pump user and understand more about insulin pump therapy.

As a pump service grows, the need for explanatory literature is also likely to grow. Policies will need to be developed for the management of insulin pumps for inpatients, for example, or for surgical procedures under general anaesthetic. It might not be necessary to develop all this literature in the initial stages of setting up a service; it might be easier to do so when more experience has been gained and ideas have developed within the team about how to manage pumps in different situations.

## RECORD-KEEPING FOR PUMP USERS

Record-keeping is important, both for health professionals and for insulin pump users. It is useful to develop specific insulin pump records to ensure that adequate information is recorded when pump users are reviewed. An example of what information health professionals' records might contain is given in Table 5.2. However, this list is not exhaustive, and there might be many additional comments and notes taken during a consultation, as with any other diabetes consultation. Having a firm framework to guide the process used within a consultation is helpful, and over time this can be adapted and flexibility increased as confidence and expertise in insulin pump therapy grows.

The records that individual pump users keep need to be as detailed as possible in the very early days of pump therapy. This makes it much easier to review the success of insulin pump therapy, for example, if they record

**Table 5.2**   Information for health professionals to record in pump users' medical records

---

*Information to record prior to starting insulin pump therapy:*
Insulin type and doses
HbA1c
Weight and body mass index (BMI)
How frequently hypoglycaemic episodes occur
Warning signs of hypoglycaemia
Existing complications, especially retinopathy
Other medical conditions
Why an insulin pump is going to be used
Any specific individual considerations

*When starting a pump:*
The type of pump and type of insulin used
The initial basal rate, and how this has been calculated
The insulin to carbohydrate ratio used
The correction dose ratio used
The type of infusion set used
Agreed blood glucose levels to aim for, both initially and in the longer term
General diabetes management targets (such as a reduction in hypoglycaemia) and timescales for achieving them
Any specific individual needs and how they are being met

*Review in the early days:*
Blood glucose readings, with dates and times
Amount and type of carbohydrate eaten
Food bolus doses given and how they were delivered
Any hypoglycaemia, what caused it and how it was managed
Any alterations made to the basal rate, including use of temporary basal rates
Any alterations made to the insulin food bolus or correction dose ratios
What blood glucose levels are now being aimed for
How specific situations such as physical activity or high blood glucose levels have been managed, how successful the management was and how it is agreed they will be managed in the future
Any specific individual needs and how they are being met

*Longer-term review:*
Total daily insulin doses
Basal rates, insulin to carbohydrate ratio and correction dose ratio being used
Infusion set use and sites, and frequency of resiting
HbA1c
Weight and BMI
Hypoglycaemia, causes and management
Ongoing blood glucose level targets
General management of lifestyle issues (physical activity, day-to-day variations)
Any specific individual needs and how they are being met

---

any short periods when the pump is removed or they have used a temporary decrease in their basal rate, this can be compared with any changes to their blood glucose readings and can help in working out what the best course of action is to manage each situation in the future. All carbohydrate intake should be recorded, both in grams of carbohydrate and also what food has been eaten, to assess the accuracy of carbohydrate assessment and how quickly different types of food are absorbed. Alterations to basal rates, what bolus doses have been given and what type of boluses were used and all blood glucose readings should be recorded, including what time different functions were carried out.

The pump user should also be encouraged to write down as much additional information as possible, for example if they have been particularly stressed, more active than usual, had a cold or other minor ailment or experienced any hypoglycaemic episodes, together with their ideas on why variations in blood glucose levels have occurred. The aim of collecting this information is to be able to identify what strategies have worked for the pump user, what situations could have been managed better (and if so how) and whether the insulin doses are adjusted to best manage their glycaemic control.

It is also important to keep track of whether target blood glucose ranges are being achieved and whether pump therapy is addressing the issues that initially led to their using a pump. For example, for someone with regular admissions to hospital for ketoacidosis, the aim might be to reduce the number of hospital admissions they have. For someone else, it might be to reduce the number of times they access emergency services to treat a hypoglycaemic episode.

On a long-term basis, most pump users will decide for themselves what written records they want to keep. They are likely to very quickly stop writing down the food they eat, might stop recording their blood glucose readings because their meter has a memory or might not record changes they have made to their basal rate. While this is because they are growing in confidence and don't need to write everything down to know whether it is working for them, when attending a clinic appointment it can be more difficult to identify what proactive management decisions might help. Developing a system or agreement with the pump user about what needs to be regularly written down, and also what information it would be useful to bring to a clinic appointment, will help ensure that the best use is made of the time. Open discussions are important at this stage, as written records are unlikely to be kept accurately unless the pump user believes they are important. If there are specific aims and targets to achieve (see the section 'Measuring the success of an insulin pump service'), record-keeping should also reflect those.

Pump users can download their pump data to help them keep computer records of how they have managed their pump. While these are useful, they need to be comprehensive, to encompass many of the details discussed in the preceding paragraphs. They can be used within a consultation to identify successes and areas that need adjustment and can also be used at home by individual pump users on a daily basis. Some pump users find this method of analysis extremely useful, but this is not a universal opinion (see Chapter Three for more information on their views).

## MEASURING THE SUCCESS OF AN INSULIN PUMP SERVICE

Within the NHS, measuring how successful or effective services or treatments are is of key importance. With new services particularly, budget-holders are looking for measurable success, and being able to provide them with information to demonstrate success is a way of ensuring ongoing funding for the service.

Identifying the criteria the diabetes specialist team and local service users feel would demonstrate success of the service is a useful starting point. The measures put in place should reflect the wishes of individuals within a team – some of these might relate to clinical improvements, some to how frequently medical services are accessed and some to quality-of-life issues.

Identifying how the PCOs will determine the success of the service is also important. Some of their criteria will be similar to those of the diabetes team and service users, but they might have additional criteria that relate to the cost-effectiveness of the treatment, for example whether reductions in inpatient stays are achieved. It is important to establish with the PCO at the outset how success will be defined, as this is likely to influence future funding. Table 5.3 lists some criteria that can be used as a starting point to measure the success of a service, although this list is not exhaustive.

## Measuring success for individual pump users

In addition to generic targets, individual targets should be set to measure the success of insulin pump therapy for each pump user. These targets are

**Table 5.3**   Examples of criteria to measure the success of a service

Each pump user with an HbA1c above 8% achieves a reduction in HbA1c of at least 0.5% within the first three months of starting to use a pump.
The reduction in HbA1c should be sustained for at least 12 months.
Individuals experiencing hypoglycaemia will have a reduced number of episodes.
Individuals who previously required frequent admission to hospital will be admitted less frequently over a 12-month period.

likely to relate to the main reasons why a pump was started, such as reducing fluctuations in blood glucose levels, gaining confidence in going out alone without fear of disabling hypoglycaemia, reducing the symptoms experienced from complications or reducing the number of days lost from work through diabetes-related difficulties.

It is also important to be clear about what situations would demonstrate that insulin pump therapy has *not* been a success for each individual. Identifying this from the outset makes decision-making easier if pump therapy needs to be discontinued. The agreement might be based on the agreed criteria for success, although some people might not achieve those criteria but gain other benefits. There might also be standard parameters that are assessed to see if the pump user has gained any benefit, such as a reduction in blood glucose fluctuations, less time off work, less time in hospital, less hypoglycaemia or a reduction in HbA1c levels, and pump users could be assessed to identify any benefits gained in these areas. It is important that a clear understanding be reached with the person with diabetes before pump therapy is started, and the measures used should be as objective as possible.

## Audit

If information is required for audit purposes, the data collected on individuals should also feed into a bigger system. This might be possible through a computer system, but specific categories of information might need to be added to the range of data within standard diabetes register packages, as indicated in the 'Record-keeping for pump users' section above. It might be possible to develop a range of options for each aspect, for example 'why the pump has been started' with a number of choices that can be ticked. If this information is not collected using a computer system, it is still possible to collect it manually, although more time-consuming. The diabetes team need to agree what information is required for audit purposes, in order to be able to integrate it into the record-keeping for people using insulin pumps. Information can be collected retrospectively but is much easier to collect on an ongoing basis, and it might be worth investing time to discuss this prior to starting an insulin pump service, or in the early days of providing the service.

On a national basis, an insulin pump clinical database has been set up at Leeds University (Department of Health, 2007). The aim of this database is to research the long-term effects of insulin pump therapy on glycaemic control, complications of diabetes and NHS costs. It is anticipated that the database will develop by collecting data from a large number of areas providing specialist insulin pump therapy services, and could form the basis for a national register of pump users.

## CONCLUSION

This chapter has discussed many different aspects of setting up a pump service, from gaining agreement within a diabetes team through many organisational aspects to measuring the success of a service. Many insulin pump services are set up without all these things in place, but as insulin pump use is more common many blueprints exist across the country regarding how a successful pump service can be run. The information in this chapter is designed to help address the stumbling blocks that might be encountered when a pump service is being developed, and the more planning that can be done in the early stages, the more robust the service will be, with less chance of funding or resources being queried or withdrawn.

## REFERENCES

Department of Health (2001) *Health and Social Care Act*, DH, London.
Department of Health (2007) *Insulin Pump Services*, DH, London.
National Institute for Health and Clinical Excellence (2003) *Guidance on the use of continuous subcutaneous insulin infusion for diabetes*, NICE, London.

# Chapter 6
# Assessing Suitability to Use an Insulin Pump

There is much debate between health professionals about how to assess people with diabetes regarding their suitability for using an insulin pump. In some specialist diabetes teams, strict selection criteria are applied, and exclusion criteria are used to identify those whom health professionals feel are less likely to succeed with this therapy. In part, this is driven by the negative experiences of the 1970s and 1980s, as discussed in Chapter One. There is also a political impetus to ensure that the therapy improves clinical outcomes: insulin pumps are viewed as an expensive treatment option in relation to other types of insulin therapy, and ongoing funding might rely on health professionals needing to continually demonstrate success. In these cases, a 'guilty till proven innocent' approach is often adopted, with people with diabetes having to 'prove' that they are able and willing to work hard and actively manage an insulin pump before being allowed access to this therapy.

At the other end of the scale, where enthusiastic health professionals have seen the benefits insulin pump therapy can bring to people with diabetes, and advocate its much wider use, there is less concern about applying very strict criteria, although detailed assessment is still undertaken. Anecdotally, health professionals working in diabetes teams with a wide experience of using insulin pumps describe how they initially used very strict criteria to select people who were allowed to use a pump. As their own confidence has grown, they have developed a much more open approach, and now use pump therapy for people they might previously have excluded. This suggests that, although a wider range of people might benefit from pump use than was previously thought, health professionals might need to gain experience and develop confidence in pump management before offering it to more people. For diabetes teams just starting to use insulin pumps, careful selection of who is suitable could be a cautious but prudent approach. In short, there is still some way to go before insulin pump therapy is seen as a real option for many people with diabetes.

This chapter will focus on the main criteria to be considered when assessing whether someone is likely to find success with using an insulin pump. Rather than providing exclusion criteria, the focus is on using a positive approach, with exclusion being applied only to those who fail to meet the criteria, although as with any clinical situation there might be justifiable exclusions when these criteria are applied in clinical practice. The examples will identify what the criteria might look like in practice. They are not in any order of priority, as they are all important.

## CLINICAL NEED

From the health professional's point of view – and of those holding the budgets to fund pump therapy – clinical need is often the first indication that pump therapy might be of benefit. There are a number of situations where this might be apparent:

## Poor glycaemic control

As NICE guidance (2003) suggests, people with high HbA1c levels who appear unable to reduce this despite optimising their insulin regimen might fit into this category. But HbA1c levels alone should not be the only marker of poor glycaemic control. For people having difficulty stabilising their blood glucose levels, and experiencing large fluctuations between blood glucose levels throughout the day and night, a pump might offer a solution. Likewise, seeing a large morning rise in blood glucose levels (commonly referred to as the 'dawn phenomenon'), which is difficult to manage using multiple-dose insulin therapy, is a clinical indication that an insulin pump might be of benefit.

## Hypoglycaemia and hypoglycaemia unawareness

Experiencing regular, severe or unpredictable hypoglycaemia is another common reason for pump use. Being able to stabilise blood glucose levels and reduce day-to-day fluctuations is likely to reduce the risk of hypoglycaemia. In those who are unaware when their blood glucose is falling, this can help restore their previous hypoglycaemia symptoms.

# Pregnancy

Poor glycaemic control in the early stages of pregnancy can result in congenital malformations and other complications, but achieving the tight control necessary prior to and during pregnancy using multiple-dose insulin therapy is likely to result in regular hypoglycaemia. An insulin pump can help pregnant women with diabetes by providing the opportunity to make more effective changes to their insulin dose as their insulin needs increase, particularly in the third trimester, and also results in better outcomes in terms of a reduced incidence of congenital malformations and stillbirths.

# Babies, children and teenagers

Pumps can be used in babies and toddlers to avoid the scenario of having to eat after insulin has been given, and to allow them to regularly snack, or 'graze', throughout the day and take their insulin accordingly without multiple injections. Adolescents can also benefit, as the erratic growth spurts and hormonal changes they experience during teenage years can be difficult to manage using other insulin delivery methods.

# Long-term complications

For those developing long-term complications of diabetes, using an insulin pump can enable them to gain tighter glycaemic control and thereby halt or slow the progression of complications. Many people who start pump therapy report a reduction in the symptoms of their complications, for example pain from peripheral neuropathy. With gastroparesis, where gastric emptying is unpredictable, insulin doses can more readily be adjusted using a pump to fit the individual's situation.

# PSYCHOLOGICAL NEED

Psychological need is more difficult to measure and assess than clinical need, as it might or might not result in clinical endpoints being affected. However, its effect on an individual can be just as devastating.

## Depression and associated conditions

Diabetes is a condition that affects emotions as well as having physical effects, and people can experience despair, failure and many other feelings related to their diabetes and whether they are able to adequately manage it. For example, many people experience a feeling of restriction in lifestyle with their diabetes, which can lead to resentment and depression. It is also likely to manifest itself in the way that people look after their diabetes: they might be less likely to test their blood glucose, make alterations to their insulin dose or proactively manage their diabetes in other ways, as they feel that nothing they do has any beneficial effect. Having an insulin pump can provide them with a way of more effectively managing their diabetes, and so help them feel in control again.

## Overtreatment of diabetes

For some people, the psychological impact of diabetes is to spend disproportionate amounts of time trying to make sense of its management, and often failing to achieve the results they are striving for. Individuals who continually test their blood glucose and adjust their insulin doses reactively are often labelled 'obsessive' by health professionals. They are usually keen to manage their diabetes well but find that even with multiple-dose insulin therapy they are unable to produce the success they want. People experiencing this type of frustration are likely to put a great deal of effort into pump management, and appreciate the benefits of being able to make precise insulin dose adjustments and see the results.

## Omission of insulin doses

Another sign of a psychological need might be that someone is omitting insulin doses from an intensive management regimen because of the inconvenience of taking insulin in some situations, although this might be viewed as mismanagement of their diabetes and therefore suggest they are unsuitable for using a pump. Finding out their thoughts on why they appear to not look after their diabetes is the first step in assessing this situation, as the reality of daily injecting and the difficulty in assessing the effectiveness of their insulin doses can lead to a feeling of not being able to succeed in their diabetes management. For some people, providing them with a tool to help them succeed, by using insulin pump therapy, can help restore their enthusiasm and commitment to managing their diabetes effectively.

## LIFESTYLE NEED

Insulin pump therapy is the treatment of choice for people whose lifestyle is restricted through using a conventional insulin regimen or whose variability of lifestyle makes it difficult to adequately adjust injected insulin doses to compensate. Lifestyle issues can be viewed as of secondary importance to clinical or psychological needs, but management using multiple-dose insulin therapy can result in unacceptable fluctuations in blood glucose levels, poor glycaemic control and hypoglycaemia. It can be argued that helping people to normalise their lives and gain good glycaemic control in these situations is not only about lifestyle but also about achieving good clinical outcomes. While it might be difficult to argue the case locally for people needing pumps to improve their lifestyle, approaching the issue from a clinical or psychological perspective should carry greater weight.

## Shift work

Insulin pump therapy can benefit someone's lifestyle when they work different shifts, particularly if their shift pattern includes night shifts or varies from one day or week to the next. Using a pump means that insulin can be adjusted to match any circumstances, whether the shift work involves night and day shifts, variation in mealtimes or unpredictable patterns of activity. Different basal rates and timings can be set for different shift patterns, and meal insulin doses can be matched more closely to the individual's needs.

## Regular physical activity

For people wishing to undertake physical activity that is likely to affect their glycaemic control, management of their diabetes is much easier using a pump. Basal insulin can be matched to insulin needs before, during and after activity, whereas with other methods of insulin delivery altering the amount of basal insulin available for a period of a few hours is not possible. Bolus doses of insulin can be adjusted around the period of activity and snacks eaten if required, although with insulin pump therapy it is possible to manage diabetes and physical activity solely through the adjustment of insulin doses rather than snacking.

## Variability in daily routines

Many people who have a lot of variability in their daily routine find that multiple-dose insulin therapy is inadequate to manage their diabetes and spend a lot of time trying to react to the different situations they find themselves in. Regular travelling is one example of this, especially long-distance flights, or unpredictability in activity at work, and an insulin pump can help them manage their diabetes in these situations more effectively.

# CAPABILITY

Part of the assessment process prior to using a pump is identifying whether an individual is capable of managing this type of therapy. This includes their intellectual capability to understand the principles of insulin pump therapy and to be able to work out how to adjust their insulin doses to suit various circumstances. It also includes physical capability, to be able to work the pump and deal with all the technical aspects of using it.

## Intellectual capability

It is important to objectively assess intellectual capability in relation to whether an individual will be able to use a pump, rather than prejudge their ability based on limited information about them, as this might mean that some people who would be able to manage and would benefit from a pump are denied the use of one (Farkas-Hirsch and Hirsch, 1994). Intellectual capability can be assessed by identifying whether someone can demonstrate understanding, possibly using a question-and-answer approach, of many aspects of pump therapy. For example, questions could be asked about the benefits they are likely to gain, the drawbacks, their understanding of how insulin can be adjusted in different circumstances and their ability to think logically when applying existing or taught knowledge to new situations.

Because pump users are required to make decisions throughout each day, and because there are nearly always a number of different ways that a situation can be managed using a pump, the assessment should focus on how they are able to apply what they know and how sound their decision-making process is, or is likely to develop in the future. Many experienced specialist diabetes teams report that pump use is increasing in groups of people who might appear challenging to teach, for example those with limited numeracy or literacy skills, and, while the input they require from health professionals might be greater than for other pump users, they can have equal success. For pump users who are dependent on others to make the decisions, for example young children or some people with psychiatric conditions, this assessment should focus on the carer as they will be playing the major part in pump management.

## Physical capability

When assessing physical capability, it is important to consider the facts and not exclude someone because they might have a little more difficulty in managing insulin pump therapy than other pump users. For example, someone who is blind might be thought to be unsuitable, but there are ways in which they can safely use an insulin pump. The audible beeps can be used to guide them when programming boluses, and back-up and support from a close family member or friend will mean there is someone who can check their technique and insulin doses from time to time and carry out the tasks that require sight, such as priming the insulin tubing and ensuring no air bubbles are present. Likewise, if someone has severe peripheral neuropathy or deformities of the hands, asking them to demonstrate how they will manage the practical handling aspects of the pump should be part of the assessment process. Encouraging a potential pump user to handle the pump prior to its use, to gain confidence in the pump's menu system, how the equipment fits together and how to programme insulin doses will help the health professional to assess whether they are capable of using a pump. Also, ensuring they have adequate support systems, from their partners, family members or others, will mean that any areas of concern can be regularly monitored.

## ENTHUSIASM

Pump therapy is unlikely to be successful if the person with diabetes isn't keen to use a pump or to learn different ways of managing their diabetes. As discussed in Chapter One, the lack of assessment of this aspect was a contributing factor to pump therapy being viewed as a failure in the 1970s. Many people who use insulin pumps are self-referred, having found out about them from others with diabetes, the Internet or elsewhere. These people might be highly enthusiastic, and while it is important to maintain their enthusiasm it is also crucial that they are not under any illusions that pump therapy simply means that the insulin pump does all the work and that they understand that they have a very important part to play in contributing to the success of the therapy.

There might also be people who are identified as potentially benefiting from a pump from a clinical or other point of view but who might initially be unenthusiastic and apprehensive about making such a radical change to their insulin regimen. These people might need to try insulin pump therapy for a few weeks or months initially, to be able to make an informed decision about whether it is the right therapy for them.

Regular blood glucose testing and adjusting insulin doses are daily activities when using a pump. It is important for health professionals not to prejudge someone regarding how much effort they will put into managing pump therapy on the basis of their current self-management, such as infrequent blood glucose testing. A lack of regular blood testing is common among people with diabetes, for many different reasons, such as being unable to control blood glucose levels or becoming dispirited or depressed about continual high readings.

If someone is not testing frequently, it is important to find out what their personal reasons are and to assess with them their potential for more frequent blood glucose testing and insulin adjustment if they start to use pump therapy. In most areas, people are encouraged to attend carbohydrate-counting and insulin adjustment education sessions prior to considering insulin pump therapy, to prepare them in advance and also identify whether they have the commitment, or desire, to manage their diabetes in a more intensive way. Looking at whether individuals are able to regularly test their blood following attendance at these sessions, and to make changes based on the results, can help the health professional assess whether they are likely to do so when using a pump. Whether or not this option is available, having open discussions with them about their reasons for not testing, and asking them to identify how frequently they are likely to test using insulin pump therapy, can form part of the pre-pump assessment. Care needs to be taken to avoid labelling people as 'unmotivated' or 'non-compliant' in relation to the self-management of their diabetes; instead, their reasons for their self-management decisions should be explored.

## ADDITIONAL CONSIDERATIONS PRIOR TO PUMP USE

There are a number of other considerations that might affect whether an insulin pump would be suitable for someone.

## Optimising multiple-dose insulin therapy

One aspect that should be part of the pre-pump assessment is whether an individual's multiple-dose insulin therapy has been optimised. For example, they might be sticking to a very rigid routine with their current therapy and so could gain benefit from being more flexible in adjusting their insulin doses to match their lifestyle. The Type 1 diabetes education programmes available in most localities help to address this, by teaching people how to more closely match their insulin doses to their food. Many people find that attending one of these programmes helps them to manage their diabetes well enough without needing to switch to using an insulin pump.

## Lipohypertrophy

Lipohypertrophy is a common reason why many people experience erratic glycaemic control. If they are continually injecting into lumpy injection sites, their insulin will not be working effectively. Simply altering the site where they inject their insulin can improve their glycaemic control and the predictability of the effect of their insulin. This point is an example of what might seem a basic or obvious intervention, but changes of injection sites should be explored as a potential remedy for erratic control. A significant number of individuals find that by using different injection sites they can continue their usual insulin delivery method with improved outcomes and do not need to convert to insulin pump therapy.

## Eating disorders

Insulin pump therapy could be considered an inappropriate choice for someone with an eating disorder or with a psychological condition that alters their perspective on life, as they might try to use insulin pump therapy as a tool to manipulate their diabetes and gain attention. However, in this example, dietary 'rules' being imposed on them because of their diabetes, possibly at a young age, might have been a contributing factor to their developing an eating disorder. Assessing whether the individual has insight into their difficulties and is willing to work in partnership, for example by attending an eating disorders clinic, can help in the pre-pump assessment process. As pump therapy provides a method of insulin delivery that allows people to have a real choice of whether they eat or not, for some it might provide a positive step towards treating their eating disorder.

## Psychiatric disorders

In situations where there is evidence of someone having disordered thought processes or there is the suspicion that there might be some psychological disturbance or manipulation, more thorough psychological or psychiatric assessment by trained staff is required to assess their suitability for insulin pump therapy. It is prudent in this type of situation to approach using an insulin pump very cautiously, and many specialist teams involve psychologists in their insulin pump assessment process for this reason.

## CONCLUSION

This chapter has explored many different ways that individuals can be assessed prior to using insulin pump therapy. Continuity and consistency in the approach to this within the diabetes team will help to ensure that adequate assessment is carried out on each individual and will also be a more transparent process that can stand up to examination if necessary, for example if someone is assessed as not suitable and wishes to challenge that decision. Developing criteria and agreeing how they will be assessed is one of the core recommendations when developing a specialist insulin pump service, as discussed in Chapter Five.

## REFERENCES

Farkas-Hirsch R, Hirsch IB (1994) Continuous subcutaneous insulin infusion: A review of the past and its implementation for the future. *Diabetes Spectrum* **7**(2): 80–138.
National Institute for Health and Clinical Excellence (2003) *Guidance on the use of continuous subcutaneous insulin infusion for diabetes*, NICE, London.

# Chapter 7
# Matching Insulin Doses to Carbohydrate Intake

One part of successful pump therapy management includes the accurate assessment of carbohydrate intake, in order that insulin doses can be closely matched to the individual's needs. This chapter looks at why carbohydrate assessment is important, how it has been used in the past and how that relates to current carbohydrate assessment. It identifies what information pump users need and provides help on how to assess not only the carbohydrate content of food but also other factors that will influence blood glucose levels and insulin requirements, such as different food types and alcohol intake. It then discusses how insulin doses can be calculated and when different types of boluses might be needed in different situations. Lastly, it provides guidance on how to approach educating someone with diabetes about assessing their carbohydrate intake and what ongoing follow-up they are likely to need. To be able to help someone with diabetes learn how to assess their carbohydrate intake, carbohydrate-counting reference lists will be needed in addition to the information in this chapter.

## AN INTRODUCTION TO CARBOHYDRATE ASSESSMENT

Of all the insulin therapies available, insulin delivery using a pump is the one that most closely resembles the physiological production of insulin. This does not happen automatically, however, and the pump user has to try and match the doses of insulin they programme into the pump with their body's insulin needs. Specific amounts of carbohydrate will raise someone's blood glucose by a certain amount on a repeated basis – for most people, around 10 grams of carbohydrate will result in their blood glucose rising by 2–3 mmol/l (millimoles per litre). Assessing carbohydrate is an important aspect of this, as it helps the pump user anticipate what impact carbohydrate will have on their blood glucose level, and therefore how they can programme their pump to deliver insulin to closely match the expected rise in their blood glucose.

If carbohydrates are not assessed accurately, the pump user might frequently need to give additional correction boluses after meals to deal with hyperglycaemia, or conversely they might experience hypoglycaemia if the mealtime insulin dose is too large. Helping a pump user become confident in assessing their carbohydrate intake is one of the key roles of health professionals.

## The history of carbohydrate assessment

Carbohydrate assessment has been used in diabetes management in a number of different ways in the past. This has contributed to some of the lingering myths that are still perpetuated today, particularly in relation to the need to restrict carbohydrate intake.

When less was known about diabetes and before the discovery of insulin, it was believed that, because diabetes was related to the metabolism of carbohydrate, reducing the amount of carbohydrate eaten was the obvious treatment (Bliss, 1982). Even after insulin became available, strict, carbohydrate-limited diets were still viewed as an essential part of diabetes treatment. As recently as 20 years ago, recommendations still existed for newly diagnosed people with diabetes to be 'prescribed' a specific amount of carbohydrate to eat for each meal and snack, in the belief that this would help to stabilise their diabetes (Connor and Boulton, 1989).

In the 1980s, prescribed amounts of carbohydrate were replaced with the recommendation that people with diabetes should simply follow a healthy-eating plan, in line with recommendations for people without diabetes. These recommendations continued until less than a decade ago, when structured education courses for people with Type 1 diabetes started to be introduced into the United Kingdom, which once again recommended carbohydrate assessment. However, these programmes do not suggest that carbohydrate should be restricted: the aim is for people with Type 1 diabetes to be able to adjust their insulin doses in relation to the amount of carbohydrate they wish to eat. Coupled with the development of rapid-acting analogue insulins, which have a more physiological action than soluble insulins, people with diabetes can now closely match their insulin doses to their carbohydrate intake.

# Carbohydrate assessment when using insulin pump therapy

As with multiple-dose insulin therapy, carbohydrate intake is assessed in order to closely match bolus insulin doses to food intake when using insulin pump therapy. With injections, there are still some limits to the flexibility this brings. For example, someone might take an increased dose of insulin at breakfast time to account for their mid-morning snack, but they then have no choice but to eat that snack to avoid hypoglycaemia. Conversely, if no additional insulin has been taken and a snack is eaten, the individual will experience some hyperglycaemia unless they give themselves an additional injection. With a pump, extra insulin can be given at the touch of a button, so the pump user can decide what they want to eat at any time and give insulin as required.

Because the emphasis is on insulin adjustment rather than dietary restriction, people using insulin pumps should be able to eat anything they like and give insulin to match their food. There is a certain amount of anxiety among health professionals about 'allowing' people to eat what they want, as it can conjure up visions of people eating huge amounts of unhealthy food. Pump users often report that they try out different foods when they first start using a pump: 'I avoided that type of food before because I could never control my blood glucose', whereas they find that using a pump can help them manage their blood glucose better. For others, the flexibility of being able to eat less, or miss a meal completely, and still get good glycaemic control is a major benefit. Anecdotally, people report eating less sweet foods as they have less hypoglycaemic episodes to treat.

The following sections describe the different areas that need to be covered when providing education about carbohydrate assessment. The long-term aim is for people to be able to accurately assess their carbohydrate intake in most situations, and to successfully manage their blood glucose levels by taking the appropriate amount of insulin.

# Learning which foods contain carbohydrate

Helping someone develop a basic grasp of the foods that contain carbohydrate is the first step towards understanding the differing insulin requirements of different foods. The term 'carbohydrate' is probably familiar to some; others might be more familiar with 'sugars' and 'starches'. All types of carbohydrate need to be included in estimations.

Foods that are commonly known to contain carbohydrate are shown in Table 7.1, and these foods can in general be easy to identify in meals. With other

**Table 7.1**   Common sources of carbohydrate

| |
|---|
| Bread |
| Potatoes |
| Cereals |
| Rice and pasta |
| Flour and pastry products |
| Beans and pulses |
| Fruit and fruit juice |
| Milk and milk-based foods |
| Biscuits |
| Cakes |
| Sweets and chocolate |
| Desserts/puddings |

foods, it can be difficult to identify how much carbohydrate they contain, and their carbohydrate content can sometimes be ignored. These include:

- thickened liquids (e.g. sauces, gravies and soups)
- salad dressings
- sausages
- foods coated in breadcrumbs
- home-cooked foods with flour or sugar added
- ketchups and other table sauces.

Some foods that contain small amounts of carbohydrate, for example vegetables such as carrots and parsnips, are unlikely to make a difference to someone's blood glucose level unless eaten in very large quantities. Vegetables with a higher carbohydrate content, such as peas and sweetcorn, could affect blood glucose levels significantly and need insulin boluses to accompany them.

When less than five grams of carbohydrate is eaten as a meal or snack, insulin is unlikely to be needed, because of the relatively small impact this will have on blood glucose levels. An example of this is a cup of tea with milk, for most people the amount of milk added to the tea will be quite small, so insulin would not be required, whereas for a full glass of milk it would.

## ASSESSING CARBOHYDRATE CONTENT IN PRACTICE

There are a number of different methods that can be adopted to identify the amount of carbohydrate being eaten, which are discussed in the remainder of this section.

## Carbohydrate-counting books, tables and leaflets

Lists of carbohydrate-containing foods are a common source of information used by people with diabetes. There are a large number of tables, books and leaflets available; some are provided by the pump manufacturers; others can be bought in bookshops or ordered via the Internet, and in many areas specialist diabetes dietitians develop their own materials for local use. It is important to understand exactly what information is being provided, as books and leaflets can be in different formats. Information can be provided as:

- the amount of carbohydrate per 100 grams in weight of the food
- the amount of food needed to make up a 10-gram portion of carbohydrate (although some tables, especially American ones, are in 15-gram portions)
- the amount of carbohydrate in an individual portion of food (e.g. a particular biscuit, a slice of bread or a piece of fruit)
- the amount of carbohydrate in a 'normal' serving (e.g. a takeaway meal).

Additionally, it is necessary to identify whether the carbohydrate content relates to the food before or after it is cooked, and also not to confuse the weight of the food in grams with the number of grams of carbohydrate it contains. It is important to help the pump user find information they can understand and use easily, and to ensure that they are clear about exactly what size of portion, weight of food or amount of carbohydrate the information is referring to. This could mean that different people choose to use different materials: helping them to experiment with different resources, and to try and work out the carbohydrate content of the foods they usually eat, will help them to find the system that works best for them.

For people who have limited literacy and numeracy skills, or for those who simply prefer this method, pictorial representations on leaflets can help people identify how much carbohydrate they are eating, related in particular to the portion size they choose. Pictures can be incorporated into locally produced leaflets, and resources could also be developed for use in education sessions.

## Reading food labels

Food labels can provide a helpful guide to assessing carbohydrate content, particularly in relation to specific brands, as carbohydrate tables are often only average values. Labels provide the following in relation to carbohydrate:

- the amount of carbohydrate per 100 grams of the food
- how much of the total carbohydrate is sugar

- the total amount of carbohydrate per serving, an amount which is specified on the packet
- how much of the carbohydrate per serving is sugar.

When assessing carbohydrate intake from food labels, the *total* amount of carbohydrate should always be used, not just the 'sugars'. It is also important, for example with rice or pasta, to check whether the carbohydrate content relates to the weight of the food before or after it is cooked. If using the 'per serving' guide, the serving size needs to match the amount eaten; if the amount eaten is larger, the amount of carbohydrate will increase in proportion.

## Using weights and measures

For someone new to carbohydrate assessment, weighing and measuring foods will help them to become familiar with the foods they commonly eat. Finding out the weight of food will provide information for the pump user to calculate the carbohydrate content themselves by comparing with values from food tables. It is also possible to obtain weighing scales that can provide the carbohydrate content of many common foods as well as their weight.

Other methods of measuring include using measuring cups and spoons or specific cups or bowls at home to measure a known amount, for example with rice, pasta or cereals. Pump users need to get used to visually assessing food and having a general idea of how much carbohydrate it contains based on their usual eating habits, but it can still be useful for them to check the accuracy of their assessment occasionally in the longer term, particularly if their glycaemic control deteriorates over time. Some people have their own sets of measures, such as measuring spoons, that they use regularly to assess their carbohydrate intake; others prefer to estimate the amounts visually.

## Measuring carbohydrates in portions or in grams alone

Many of the structured education programmes for people with Type 1 diabetes in the United Kingdom use a system of portions – often referred to as 'CPs' (carbohydrate portions) – to assess the carbohydrate content of food, and then match insulin doses to these. A CP would be a set amount of carbohydrate – usually 10 grams, although in some countries it is more common to use 15-gram portions. The number of CPs in a meal would then be totalled up and insulin given accordingly, based on a predetermined ratio. The

**Table 7.2** Different methods of calculating meal carbohydrate values

| Calculations based on carbohydrate portions (CPs) | Calculations based on grams of carbohydrate |
|---|---|
| 2 thin slices bread = 2 CPs | 2 thin slices bread = 20 grams |
| 179 ml unsweetened orange juice = 1.5 CPs | 179 ml unsweetened orange juice = 15 grams |
| 200 ml glass of milk = 1 CP | 200 ml glass of milk = 10 grams |
| Total = 4.5 CPs | Total = 45 grams of carbohydrate |

alternative method is to measure the total grams of carbohydrate in each type of food and add them together to find the total amount. Table 7.2 provides examples of calculating the carbohydrate content of a meal using either of these methods.

Some people find it easier to work in CPs, and if their insulin to carbohydrate ratio is a straightforward calculation, such as one unit of insulin per CP, it is relatively simple to calculate. Others prefer adding up the grams of carbohydrate in their foods, and this method can be helpful if their insulin to carbohydrate ratio is more complex, for example one unit of insulin for every seven grams of carbohydrate. Some insulin pumps have a feature to calculate the insulin bolus required (further information is available in Chapter Four).

# Rounding totals up or down

When assessing carbohydrate content, pump users are generally encouraged to round the amount of carbohydrate up or down if it is not divisible by five, to enable calculation of the bolus dose. For example, 24 grams would be rounded up to 25 grams, and 42 grams would be rounded down to 40 grams. If CPs are used, as in the previous section, the grams are rounded up or down *prior* to being added together. An alternative method is to identify the exact carbohydrate content of individual foods, add them together and then round the total up or down.

Using different methods can result in different totals being reached for the same meal, as shown in Table 7.3. This does not mean that one method of calculation is superior to another; as can be seen from the example, both methods result in total carbohydrate values within five grams of each other, and both will result in an amount of insulin being given that closely relates to the amount needed. As discussed earlier in this chapter, helping the pump user find out how to consistently calculate their carbohydrate intake and insulin dose, and testing it out using their blood glucose readings as a guide, is the key to success.

**Table 7.3**   Different methods of totalling the carbohydrate content of a meal

| Calculations based on carbohydrate portions (CPs) | Calculations based on grams of carbohydrate |
| --- | --- |
| Item A = 13 grams = 1.5 CPs | Item A = 13 grams |
| Item B = 14 grams = 1.5 CPs | Item B = 14 grams |
| Item C = 28 grams = 3.0 CPs | Item C = 28 grams |
| Item D = 36 grams = 3.5 CPs | Item D = 36 grams |
| Total = 9.5 CPs | Total = 91 grams = rounded down to 90 grams |

# ACCOUNTING FOR ALCOHOL

The carbohydrate content of alcohol needs to be treated differently from that in food because of the potential for alcohol to cause hypoglycaemia a number of hours later. Identifying which types of alcohol a pump user likes to drink, and in what quantities, is a good starting point. The next step is to determine how much carbohydrate their preferred alcoholic beverages contain – most wines (unless very sweet) contain very little carbohydrate, nor do spirits, whereas beer, lager, cider and some alcopops can contain fairly substantial amounts of carbohydrate. As with carbohydrate-counting tables for food, using accurate tools for assessing the carbohydrate content of alcohol is important.

Identifying the effect alcohol has had on blood glucose levels in the past, and how it has been managed, will help individuals to identify what action they should take when using an insulin pump. Alcoholic beverages that contain carbohydrate will usually cause an initial rise in their blood glucose levels. An insulin bolus can be given to counteract that rise, but it is important to be cautious with insulin doses at this point because blood glucose levels are likely to drop a few hours later. If someone wishes to give insulin to avoid that initial hyperglycaemia, they should be encouraged to only give boluses for the first two drinks, when their blood glucose level is still rising. If they drink more than two drinks, they should omit any further boluses.

Helping a pump user understand that around 50 per cent of the glucose in their bloodstream is converted from stored glycogen in their liver and that the release of this glucose is impaired when they are drinking alcohol will help them to understand why their blood glucose level is likely to fall after more than a drink or two containing alcohol. From this, they can identify strategies to counteract that drop in their blood glucose level, to prevent hypoglycaemia. Snacking at the same time as drinking alcohol is one option, remembering *not* to give an insulin bolus for the snacks. Having a carbohydrate-rich supper before going to bed is another option, again without giving an insulin bolus. Both of these options are commonly used by people treated with multiple-dose insulin therapy.

Altering the insulin doses being delivered by the pump is another option. A temporary reduction in the basal rate can be programmed for overnight, and this can be used instead of, or in addition to, snacking. If the temporary basal rate option is chosen, it will be safer to programme this earlier in the evening rather than when under the influence of alcohol. Avoiding hypoglycaemia is the most important aspect, so over-snacking, or reducing the insulin dose too much, is a safe route initially. As the pump user gains confidence in their usual blood glucose pattern after drinking alcohol, they can then more closely estimate how much extra food and/or how much of a reduction in their insulin dose they will need.

For some people, the prolonged hypoglycaemia effect of alcohol can continue into the next day, so, as well as the measures described above, they might need to take a reduced amount of insulin at breakfast time to avoid mid-morning hypoglycaemia. Again, using their previous experience and their blood testing results will help determine the best course of action.

# EATING AWAY FROM HOME

It can be difficult to estimate the carbohydrate content of foods when eating away from home (in restaurants, at picnics and parties) or in takeaway food. Some restaurants or fast-food outlets can provide information on the carbohydrate content of foods, and some carbohydrate-counting tables give specific information about the expected carbohydrate content of foods such as fish and chips, but the portion sizes can vary enormously with this type of food. Learning how to assess foods visually and estimate their carbohydrate content takes time and effort, and blood glucose testing is vital to be able to understand more about the effects of different foods.

It can be easy for the pump user to restrict themselves to only visiting certain restaurants or eating certain types of foods, but it is more useful to have a general plan of how to deal with foods where the carbohydrate content is uncertain. Deciding how much carbohydrate is likely to be in the food, and giving possibly a smaller than anticipated bolus, is the safest way as this will help to avoid hypoglycaemia. If this method is used, a correction ratio might be needed a couple of hours later, so blood glucose levels should always be checked to determine this. Having small boluses for different courses of a meal, or when snacking at a party, also helps the insulin to more closely match the food eaten.

# WORKING OUT INSULIN TO CARBOHYDRATE RATIOS

Identifying how much insulin someone needs to take to match their food when first starting to use a pump, and getting it right, can be difficult. In most specialist diabetes teams, a standard ratio of one unit of insulin to 10 grams of carbohydrate (1 CP) is used as a starting point. It is important to recognise that this might not be the ratio that suits everyone, although anecdotally it is likely to be close to the needs of the majority of pump users.

If someone has already been adjusting their insulin in relation to the food they eat, so they already have an insulin to carbohydrate ratio that works for them, they might wish to continue using this ratio in the first instance, although it might need altering if hypoglycaemia is occurring. Over time, the insulin to carbohydrate ratio can then be reviewed and adapted if required.

There can be times when the insulin to carbohydrate ratio is increased or decreased from the outset, depending on the individual's situation. For example, if someone appears to need very small amounts of insulin prior to starting to use a pump, they might need less insulin for their food boluses, so one unit to 20 grams could be used. At the other end of the scale, people with a high level of insulin resistance, for example those who are very overweight, might need a larger amount of insulin, although evidence suggests that insulin resistance can be combated most effectively by delivering insulin using a pump, which could result in less insulin being needed (Pouwels *et al.*, 2003).

Another option for calculating someone's insulin to carbohydrate ratio is to use the '500 rule'. This is a calculation based on the total amount of insulin taken over a 24-hour period. The number 500 is divided by the total daily insulin dose, and the answer indicates how much carbohydrate will match one unit of insulin. If this equation is used when pump therapy is first initiated, the calculation should be based on the pre-pump total daily dose minus the percentage reduction (usually 30 per cent) and before dividing the total by two to establish the basal rate. Table 7.4 provides examples of how the calculations work.

**Table 7.4**  Calculating insulin to carbohydrate ratios using the 500 rule

---

Total daily insulin dose = 50 units
500/50 = 10
So 1 unit of insulin = 10 grams of carbohydrate (or 1 unit per CP)

Total daily insulin dose = 25 units
500/25 = 20
So 1 unit of insulin = 20 grams of carbohydrate (or 0.5 units per CP)

---

One of the drawbacks of using the 500 rule when insulin pump therapy is being initiated is that using someone's pre-pump insulin dose is unlikely to be a good indicator of how much insulin they will need when using a pump, particularly in situations where their glycaemic control has been less than optimal. Calculating their insulin to carbohydrate ratio in this way could result in a less accurate assessment of their insulin to carbohydrate ratio. Most diabetes teams experienced in pump use are more likely to use the standard one unit to 10 grams of carbohydrate as a starting point. However, the 500 rule is useful when reviewing progress, as it can provide a rough guide of what ratio is likely to be effective.

## WHICH TYPE OF BOLUS TO USE

Once the carbohydrate content of a meal or snack has been established, and the amount of insulin has been decided, the pump user needs to decide what type of bolus to give, whether a standard bolus, extended or mixed bolus is required. Even before learning how to assess their carbohydrate intake, many people with Type 1 diabetes can identify specific foods or types of meals that cause a prolonged rise in their blood glucose level, which can be a good guide to their rate of absorption of different foods and so help with their choice of which insulin bolus to use.

Chapter 10 provides a more detailed explanation of the different types of bolus and the terms used to describe them. To identify the type of bolus that is appropriate for a specific situation, helping a pump user understand what factors affect the absorption of the carbohydrate they are eating, as listed in Table 7.5, will help them closely match their insulin doses to their food intake.

Foods that are absorbed more quickly are likely to need standard boluses of insulin given, whereas those that are absorbed more slowly might require a different type of bolus. Looking at the factors in Table 7.5, high-GI foods will be absorbed the fastest and so are likely to need insulin given immediately. For foods with a lower GI rating, they might need a more prolonged insulin bolus, and how to calculate this is discussed later in this chapter.

**Table 7.5**  Factors affecting the speed of absorption of carbohydrate

- Glycaemic Index (GI) rating
- Fat content
- Protein content
- Quantity of carbohydrate

**Table 7.6**  Use of different types of bolus

| Type of bolus | How insulin is delivered | Main use of this type of bolus |
|---|---|---|
| Standard | Immediately | When the total carbohydrate amount is less than 50 grams<br>When food has a high GI |
| Extended | At a constant rate over a specified number of hours | When food has a low GI<br>High-protein, high-fat or high-fibre foods<br>When more than 50 grams of carbohydrate is eaten |
| Mixed | Part immediately, part at a constant rate over a specified number of hours | When some insulin is required immediately and some over a longer period, generally in situations similar to the extended bolus use above |

A meal with a high fat content (more than 15–20 grams of fat in total in the meal) or high protein content (more than 20–30 grams of protein in total) will also slow down absorption, so a prolonged insulin bolus might be the best choice in those circumstances. It can be difficult to assess the amount of fat and protein in a meal as well as the carbohydrate content, but discussing the pump user's food preferences and usual choices can help to identify the types of foods that are likely to require more prolonged boluses.

The quantity of carbohydrate eaten in one meal also affects absorption, as larger quantities of food will take longer to digest. As a general guide, meals containing more than 50 grams of carbohydrate are likely to need a more prolonged insulin bolus. Table 7.6 provides general guidance on when the different boluses might be used, although the individual pump user's response to types and quantities of foods should always be taken into account.

As a guide, most carbohydrate-containing foods require some insulin immediately, irrespective of whether the food will have a prolonged effect on their blood glucose, so either a standard or a mixed bolus is the one most commonly chosen. Some pump users prefer to give a number of standard boluses even if their food will have a prolonged effect on their blood glucose, so they might, for example, take 70 per cent of the dose they need when they start eating and 30 per cent at a later time, probably within 60 minutes of their first dose. Splitting the bolus dose in these proportions has been shown to be effective (Chase *et al.*, 2002) and is discussed further in Chapter 10.

All the above are general principles, and the only way to assess the success of any method is by using blood glucose testing results. Pre-meal blood glucose levels and physical activity just before or after meals are additional factors that can affect what amount of insulin and type of bolus is chosen. More information on interpreting results and deciding what action to take is in Chapter 11.

## HOW TO TEACH CARBOHYDRATE ASSESSMENT

When teaching a potential pump user how to assess their carbohydrate intake, the provision of information as described in this chapter is important, but people also need help to apply what they are learning to real-life situations. Ideally, carbohydrate assessment should be taught over a number of sessions, to allow people time to experiment between sessions and to apply their growing knowledge to their own day-to-day situations. Also, as discussed in Chapter Nine, learning about carbohydrate assessment might be part of a structured education programme that is undertaken some time before initiating pump therapy.

It can be helpful to develop a number of resources, both for use in the clinic and for pump users to take away, that can be used to raise people's awareness of amounts of carbohydrate, as in the following sections.

### Food diaries

People with diabetes need to be able to apply the knowledge gained in education sessions to the specific foods they eat regularly as a starting point. Keeping food and blood glucose monitoring diaries, and bringing them to their next appointment or group session, can help them to become confident in assessing their day-to-day food, and allows them to check out their own calculations when they return.

### Food models

Being able to visualise the amounts of different foods and their carbohydrate content is helpful, for example it can be quite difficult to visually assess how much carbohydrate is in a portion of rice or mashed potato. Comparing the food models with the amount the individual normally eats can help them work out the likely carbohydrate content of their meals.

### Food labels and containers

Cereal boxes, yoghurt pots, canned foods and ready meals are all examples of foods with labels that can be used to help people understand carbohydrate content. Providing a wide variety of food labels will mean that people can identify those which they eat most commonly. It also helps them become familiar with interpreting food labels and can raise their general awareness of which foods tend to have a higher carbohydrate content. Pump users might find it useful to bring labels and containers from foods they eat at home to discuss in a consultation or education session.

## Weighing scales

Weighing carbohydrate-containing foods has already been discussed as a method of identifying the carbohydrate content of meals. Flat-topped scales are useful at home, as food can be weighed as it is served on to a plate.

## Carbohydrate reference tables and leaflets

Using books, tables and leaflets has been discussed earlier in this chapter, and having a range of different materials for use in education sessions and consultations will raise people's awareness of what resources they can use.

## Insulin dose calculators

Along with carbohydrate reference tables, many of the insulin pump manufacturers supply charts, or bolus guides, that can be used to work out the insulin dose needed for different amounts of carbohydrate. As discussed in Chapter Four, some pumps will calculate the insulin dose when the amount of carbohydrate being eaten is programmed in. If someone does not have a natural aptitude for figures, finding them the right tools that they can work with is one of the key areas of importance. Helping them use charts and pump functions to calculate insulin doses in the education sessions, either through preset exercises or by looking at the usual foods they eat, prepares them for when they need to assess carbohydrate on their own.

## Guidance about healthy eating

When discussing carbohydrates with people with diabetes, it can be seen as an opportunity to reinforce messages about eating healthily. Raising awareness of healthy food choices might be helpful, but it is important not to judge or blame people, or try and persuade them to change their eating habits, if they eat less healthy foods. If people feel criticised about their food intake, they will be less keen to be open about what they are eating. The most important thing is for people to be able to assess the carbohydrate content of *any* food they eat, so they should be encouraged to discuss less healthy foods in exactly the same way that they discuss other foods. Similarly, carbohydrate-counting tables and lists should provide information about the whole range of foods available, including those high in fat and sugar.

## Providing ongoing support and education

As with most situations, potential pump users will be eager to receive information and support when they first start to learn how to assess their carbohydrate intake, but as they become more confident they are likely to rely more on their existing knowledge and be less likely to access support from health professionals. Anecdotally, many people weigh and measure their foods much less once they have more experience and will estimate the carbohydrate content more approximately, which can sometimes result in less accuracy.

When reviewing people who have been assessing their carbohydrate intake for some time, it is helpful to talk about specific situations, such as eating out or dealing with hypoglycaemia, in order to find out how they are managing. A questioning approach – finding out when it has been difficult to assess carbohydrate content accurately, asking how they are deciding on the carbohydrate content of foods and what is working well – will help them to talk about day-to-day situations. Acknowledging the time and effort required in carbohydrate assessment, and offering support and encouragement, will help pump users feel comfortable in discussing difficulties that might account for poor glycaemic control. Celebrating successes, and helping them work out what they can do to change the situations they feel they do not manage as successfully, will help them to further develop their problem-solving skills. More information about how to use this approach in practice can be found in Chapter Eight.

## CONCLUSION

This chapter has shown why carbohydrate assessment is important, how it has been used restrictively in the management of diabetes in the past and the more helpful way it is used today. It has discussed the main carbohydrate-containing foods and also the less obvious sources of carbohydrate. It has provided guidance on how people can identify the carbohydrate content of the food they are eating and how they might need to vary the type of insulin bolus they give depending on the type and size of meal they are eating. How to approach carbohydrate assessment and insulin dosing in relation to alcohol has been discussed, along with setting an initial insulin to carbohydrate ratio; more about adjusting that ratio can be found in Chapter 10. The final part of the chapter discussed what approaches can be used when providing education about carbohydrate assessment.

As can be seen throughout the chapter, the emphasis should be on finding out what people already are aware of, and helping them reflect on what has worked in the past, as a guide to how they might manage situations using carbohydrate assessment and adjusting their insulin doses using a pump. Pump users need to be able to assess any type of food they are eating in relation to how much insulin they need, so encouraging them to experiment and work things out for themselves will strengthen their ability to do this.

## REFERENCES

Bliss M (1982) *The Discovery of Insulin*, Macmillan Press, Basingstoke.

Chase HP, Saib Z, Mackenzie T *et al.* (2002) Post prandial glucose excursions following four methods of bolus insulin administration in subjects with Type 1 diabetes. *Diabetic Medicine* **19**(4): 317–321.

Connor H, Boulton AJM (1989) *Diabetes in Practice*, John Wiley & Sons, Chichester.

Pouwels M-JJ, Tack CJ, Hermus AR, Lutterman JA (2003) Treatment with intravenous insulin followed by continuous subcutaneous insulin infusion improves glycaemic control in severely resistant Type 2 diabetic patients. *Diabetic Medicine* **20**(1): 76–79.

Chapter 8
# Using an Empowerment Approach to Insulin Pump Therapy Education

One of the important aspects of providing an insulin pump service is ensuring that people who use pumps receive adequate education to help them manage their diabetes. It has already been discussed in Chapter One that a lack of education was seen as one of the reasons why pump use failed in the 1980s in the United Kingdom. Much of the content of this book is focused on providing answers in relation to the different aspects of using insulin pump therapy, and information on all the topics discussed in this chapter can be found in other parts of this book.

This chapter will look at how education can be approached in order to maximise its effect, particularly when someone is just starting to use an insulin pump. Using a group education approach is also explored, including how the principles discussed throughout this chapter can be applied. Education needs to be thought of in its wider context, not simply as training in the technological aspects of using a pump but as a way of helping people develop coping strategies and problem-solving skills to manage their diabetes from one day to the next, no matter how different those days might be.

## THE AIMS OF EDUCATION

To be successful in providing education in relation to insulin pump therapy, the first step is to be clear about what the aims of education are. In terms of the outcomes of education, the expectations are that a pump user should be able to:

- identify what the benefits and drawbacks of using a pump are
- safely manage the technical aspects of using a pump
- accurately assess carbohydrate intake and the overall effect of different foods on glycaemic control

- work out what insulin doses to give, and what type of bolus, to match their carbohydrate intake and to treat high blood glucose levels
- successfully manage their insulin pump therapy to deal with variations in their day-to-day life
- adapt their diabetes management to address new situations
- make decisions independently (or with the help of a carer where appropriate) about all of the above.

To be able to achieve these aims, how the education is to be delivered needs to be considered. A method that simply provides information in a didactic style will meet some of the aims, for example helping someone become familiar with how to insert insulin into their pump, how to prime the tubing and what buttons to press to programme the pump. All these help towards achieving competence in the technical aspects of insulin pump management. Other information is also likely to be important, particularly in relation to the different methods of insulin delivery of a pump and new ways that insulin doses can be adjusted. While information is required, the key to success for a pump user is to be able to apply that information to the day-to-day situations they find themselves in.

For people to be able to integrate pump therapy into any situation they come across, an approach that encourages questioning and experimentation, and supports individuals to find solutions for themselves, is required. There is an abundance of evidence that the more people with diabetes are involved in discussion, negotiation and decision-making, the more likely they are to retain more information and be able to manage their diabetes more successfully (Williams *et al.*, 1998; Knight *et al.*, 2006).

## What approach should be used?

Health professionals are taught to be, and often viewed as, experts in the management of disease. The responsibilities of health professionals in this role include: finding out or diagnosing what the problem is, using their expertise to find solutions and directing the person in their care regarding what action they should take. This model works extremely well in acute care, where medical decision-making is paramount to the person receiving the right treatment to recover from an illness or situation. But it works less well with long-term conditions such as diabetes, for a number of reasons:

- There is no cure for diabetes, and any treatment does not carry the hope of someone getting better.
- There is rarely a single solution that is the correct one.

- Much of the treatment of diabetes is designed to minimise the risk of long-term complications that might or might not occur in the future.
- Many people with diabetes experience an increase in adverse symptoms when they follow health professionals' recommendations to maintain good glycaemic control.
- Whatever treatment is prescribed in diabetes, there is no guarantee that it will prevent complications developing in later life.

In addition, there is ample evidence that people with diabetes often don't follow prescribed treatment regimens. For example, it is rare for people with either Type 1 or Type 2 diabetes to follow dietary recommendations (Toobert *et al.*, 2000), and only a fifth of people taking insulin obtain enough blood glucose testing strips on prescription to test their blood glucose level even once a day (Evans *et al.*, 1999). Also, the fact that over a quarter of people with Type 1 diabetes don't obtain enough insulin on prescription to meet their requirements suggests that it is common for people to not follow treatment recommendations (Morris *et al.*, 1997). All this information lends weight to the concept that providing advice and telling people what they should do doesn't work with diabetes. To help people have more success in managing their diabetes, alternative ways need to be found to enhance people's self-care and motivation.

## AN INTRODUCTION TO EMPOWERMENT

One of the most effective ways of providing diabetes education is by using an empowerment approach (Anderson *et al.*, 1995; Lorig and Gonzalez, 1992). Standard three of the *National Service Framework for Diabetes*, 'Empowering people with diabetes', states that one of the key aims of diabetes care is to ensure that people with diabetes can 'enhance their personal control over the day to day management of their diabetes in a way that enables them to experience the best possible quality of life' (Department of Health, 2001: 21). National recommendations for providing education programmes for people with diabetes also acknowledge the key components of meeting individual needs, supporting self-management and incorporating personal choice into routine diabetes care (Department of Health, 2005; National Institute for Health and Clinical Excellence, 2003).

One of the facts underpinning the need for using an empowerment approach is that everyone has thoughts and experiences which form the basis of how they process and interpret the world around them, and these thoughts and beliefs are formed before they come to a consultation (McCann and Weinman, 1996). When we provide information to people with diabetes, they filter it, measuring it against what they already know and what they have learnt, often through experience, in the past. Even when faced with new experiences, such as being newly diagnosed with diabetes or starting to use an insulin pump, they still have beliefs, ideas and concerns that play an important part in shaping their way of dealing with the condition.

The empowerment model in diabetes was developed and researched in the United States in the 1980s and 1990s by Bob Anderson and Marti Funnell, at the University of Michigan (Funnell *et al.*, 1991; Anderson *et al.*, 1995). This model provides a five-stage process to help guide consultations. Table 8.1 outlines the five stages and provides information of what they might look like in practice within a consultation.

**Table 8.1**   The five-stage empowerment model

| | |
|---|---|
| Stage One: Identify the issue | What are you finding most difficult about your diabetes at the moment? |
| | What is the most important thing you'd like to talk about today? |
| | Can you tell me more about that? |
| | Are there some specific examples you can give me? |
| Stage Two: Explore feelings and values | What thoughts do you have about this? |
| | When (the situation) happens, how does it make you feel? |
| | You sound (angry, frightened, upset) about this – is that how it makes you feel? |
| Stage Three: Identify possible actions | How would the situation need to change for you to feel better about it? |
| | Where would you like to be with this in (suggest timescale: a few weeks/six months/a year)? |
| | What could you do to help sort this out? |
| | Are there any other things you could do? |
| | Are there any barriers to what you want to do? |
| | If so, what could you do to overcome the barriers? |
| | How important is it (on a scale of 1–10) for you to do something about this? |
| Stage Four: Commit to action | What are the first steps to take towards achieving your goals? |
| | What exactly are you going to do? |
| | When are you going to start? |
| | If you try and do this and meet any of your barriers, what will you do? |
| Stage Five: Evaluate | How did it go? |
| | What worked well for you? |
| | What didn't work so well? |
| | What thoughts have you got about what you might do next time you're in that situation? |

This model provides a framework to help move away from a didactic, advice-giving approach. However, as in diabetes, any behaviour change is difficult, and it can be hard to change health professionals' well-learnt and long-practised method of using the acute care approach, as discussed earlier in this chapter. Using the empowerment model, the health professional becomes much more of a facilitator, using open questions to take someone with diabetes through a process to help them reflect on their own knowledge, rather than the health professional having to be the expert and provide all the answers. It also helps people with diabetes to develop their decision-making capabilities around how to adapt their diabetes management to the differing situations they might find themselves in. Table 8.2 highlights the differences between a consultation using the traditional didactic approach (as taught in much of health professionals' training) and one using an empowerment approach.

**Table 8.2**  Differences between a didactic and an empowering approach to education

| Didactic | Empowering |
| --- | --- |
| The health professional identifies what the problems or issues are. | The person with diabetes is invited to identify what their problems or issues are. |
| Information is provided on the basis of what the health professional has identified as being needed. | Information is provided on the basis of what the individual needs, identified through questioning and discussion. |
| The health professional provides answers to all the questions asked by the person with diabetes. | The health professional encourages the person with diabetes to reflect on their own situation and knowledge, and to identify their own solutions to the questions they ask. |
| The health professional provides advice on what to do in different situations. | The person with diabetes is asked what they think they should do in different situations, with the health professional providing information only as a supplement. |
| The health professional decides what the person should do to manage their diabetes following the consultation. | The health professional helps the person with diabetes to make a firm plan, based on their own ideas, of what they are going to do to manage their diabetes following the consultation. |
| The responsibility lies with the health professional to sort the situation out. | The responsibility lies with the person with diabetes to manage the situation. |
| Any success in diabetes management is attributed to the health professional's decisions. | Any success in diabetes management is attributed to the decisions made by the person with diabetes. |

## Relating empowerment to insulin pump therapy

For those using insulin pumps, the empowerment model fits ideally. Many people using insulin pumps have had years of experience of managing their diabetes (although pumps are being used much earlier in some circumstances), and their experience can be used to facilitate their learning about how to use their insulin pump to manage their diabetes. For example, people will already have developed their own strategies for how they manage their diabetes in different circumstances, such as when undertaking physical activity, eating out or having a drink with friends. These strategies can be discussed, including how successful they have been, and be used to plan how best to manage those situations using insulin pump therapy. Someone who hasn't used insulin pump therapy before will need new information, but much of this should relate to how insulin doses can be given using a pump and what effect the different ways of giving insulin are likely to have. Health professionals should aim to convey information pertinent to a pump user's specific needs rather than trying to give them all the information that exists on any given subject.

## PUTTING IT INTO PRACTICE

This section provides examples of conversations that could be held with people with diabetes around a number of pump-related situations. They do not cover every issue that will be encountered but show how the principle of using an empowerment approach can be put into practice. In any of the situations described, additional information might need to be provided before the pump user can respond.

## Prior to using a pump

When someone is first thinking about using an insulin pump, or it has been suggested to them, using an empowerment approach provides the opportunity to elicit their thoughts and beliefs about insulin pump therapy. Their pre-existing ideas are likely to affect whether they have a realistic view of pump therapy and whether it will be useful to them. The individual should be encouraged to identify for themselves why they think a pump will benefit them, what they feel about it and what concerns they have, with information being supplied on the basis of a person's individual needs. Questions that could be asked by the health professional include:

- What is happening at the moment with your diabetes that you think will be helped by using an insulin pump?
- What do you think the advantages of using a pump will be for you?
- What will the drawbacks of using a pump be for you?
- What concerns do you have about insulin pump therapy?
- What would help you to feel better about this situation?
- What information can I help you with to be able to make up your mind as to whether you want to use a pump?

## Assessing carbohydrate intake

When someone is starting to learn about assessing carbohydrate intake, reflecting on what they already know, what they like and want to eat and how they are going to deal with practical issues about assessing carbohydrate can be helpful. Questions might include:

- What are the foods that you eat, or know of, that contain carbohydrate?
- What is your day like regarding what you eat and when?
- What would be an ideal pattern of what you eat and when?
- How might you work out how much carbohydrate is in the foods you are eating?
- What situations do you regularly encounter where you might find it difficult to estimate your carbohydrate intake (and how could you deal with these)?

## Working out where and how to wear the insulin pump

For some, concerns about how and where the pump will be worn can cause anxiety and negative thoughts about pump use. Encouraging the individual to think through different situations in their lives and identify the most convenient method of wearing their pump for each will help to deal with some of those anxieties. Questions might include:

- What concerns do you have about wearing your pump?
- How do you think you will normally wear your pump?
- Will you have any difficulties with this?

- What situations can you think of when you'll need to do something different?
- What do you think you might do in those circumstances?

## Deciding what amount of insulin to give

People using insulin pump therapy need to learn what standard doses of insulin they should use to match specified amounts of carbohydrate and to correct high blood glucose levels. They also need to be able to visualise what they will actually do in their day-to-day lives. Understanding how the pump works and how insulin is delivered using the different functions is important, and questions can then help them determine how they will apply that information to successfully manage their diabetes. Questions might include:

- If you are eating food containing carbohydrate, how will you work out how much insulin to give?
- In what situations will you vary that amount of insulin?
- What other factors will influence how much insulin you give?
- How will you decide if your bolus doses are working for you?
- In what situations might you think about using other types of boluses?
- Can you give me an example of when you might use something other than a standard bolus?
- How will you assess whether your basal insulin rate is working?
- If you need to alter your basal rate, how will you do that?

## Deciding how frequently to monitor blood glucose levels

The frequency of blood glucose monitoring required to manage insulin pump therapy successfully requires commitment and hard work by the pump user. This should include helping the individual work out what they know about blood glucose monitoring and how they can use it to assess their glycaemic control. Using this information in combination with knowing how the pump delivers insulin, they will be able to develop a plan of how much testing will give them enough information to make proactive decisions about managing their diabetes using an insulin pump. Questions might include:

- How frequently do you feel you need to monitor your blood glucose levels on a pump?
- What are your reasons for deciding that?

- What information do you need about your blood glucose levels to help you manage your diabetes?
- How will you use your monitoring to alert you to whether you need to make any changes?
- What readings would you consider high enough to give some extra insulin?
- In what situations will you monitor more frequently, and why?
- Is there anything that will get in the way of you monitoring as much as you have said you'd like to?
- If so, what could you do when faced with those situations?

## Working out how to deal with drinking alcohol

Where individuals are dealing with lifestyle issues that are likely to affect their glycaemic control, knowing how the pump delivers insulin and then applying their previous experiences will help them identify what management options they have. Questions might include:

- What changes have you previously made to keep yourself safe when drinking alcohol?
- What effect have those changes had? (Have they been successful? What happened as a result of what you did?)
- Now that you have a pump, what ideas do you have about what you could do to manage your diabetes when you drink alcohol?

## Working out how to deal with a physical activity regimen

Identifying what type of physical activity the individual is planning to do, and what their previous experiences have been regarding the best way of managing their diabetes at the time, will help them develop a logical plan to try out. Because the pump offers a number of different ways that insulin doses can be reduced effectively, the pump user will have more options of how they can adapt their insulin doses to physical activity than previously. Questions might include:

- What sort of activities do you do?
- How have you previously managed these situations? (What have you done with your insulin? Have you eaten extra food? If so, what?)
- What options do you have for managing your diabetes in these situations now you have an insulin pump?
- What do you think might work best for you?

- Will you need to plan anything in advance?
- What are you going to do the next time you do the activity you described?
- How will you assess whether your actions have been successful?

## Identifying how to treat a hypoglycaemic episode

This should include using the individual's previous experience, reflecting on how well their strategies for dealing with hypoglycaemia worked and helping them think through what they might do differently now that they have a different (and potentially easier to manage) method of insulin delivery. Questions might include:

- How have you treated hypoglycaemia in the past, before you had a pump?
- What has worked well, and what hasn't been so successful?
- Now that you have the pump and only quick-acting insulin, is there anything you might do differently?
- If yes, can you describe what you might do?
- How will you decide whether your strategies have been successful?
- How low will your blood glucose need to be before you decide to treat it?
- What are you going to do the next time your blood glucose drops too low?
- How will you assess whether your actions have been successful?

## Frequency of contact in the early days

Frequent contact with health professionals in the early days of using a pump is often seen as beneficial by people with diabetes, but should be negotiated. Discussing how frequently the pump user feels that contact will be useful will help them reflect on how confident they feel in making decisions about their pump management, and can help in negotiating how much help and support they need in the early days. It is also useful to discuss how they will manage their pump and what experimenting they might carry out between appointments. Questions might include:

- What do you need to try out in relation to managing your pump after you leave here today?
- What situations do you need to plan for before we meet again?
- How much time do you need to experiment before we meet (or have contact) again?
- What sort of support from me is going to be most useful?
- What situations will you find difficult to make decisions about?

- What will you do if you come across a difficult situation and have to make decisions?
- What difficulties might you encounter before we next meet, and what could you do if they happen?

## Ongoing pump management

When people start to gain some experience with using their pump, they might need help to identify strategies that have worked well or less well for them. This approach focuses mainly on reflection, exploration of experiences so far and building on what has already been learnt. It includes using a problem-solving approach to think of new and better ways of managing situations, as well as working out potential solutions to new situations. Questions might include:

- What have been your biggest difficulties in managing your diabetes and your pump?
- What have you done to deal with these?
- What could you have done differently?
- What are you going to do the next time these situations occur?
- What has worked well for you?
- Which of your blood glucose readings are you happy with?
- What do you think caused the readings you are not happy with?
- What could you do to get more of the blood glucose readings you want?
- What are the main things you are going to do when you leave here?

## Summary of putting it into practice

The above are all examples of discussions that could be held that are specific to the issues highlighted, but are not exclusive. As illustrated, this approach uses questioning by the health professional as the method of drawing out what the pump user thinks and feels, and what they might do as a result. It relies on previous experiences as well as current thoughts and encourages a proactive management of insulin pump therapy and troubleshooting in advance of difficult situations occurring. It does not take the place of ensuring that people with diabetes have correct information on which they are basing their decisions, and part of a health professional's duty is to correct misbeliefs and misinformation, particularly related to safety issues, such as the management of alcohol and diabetes. The scenarios discussed here are a sample of the type of issues that are likely to be discussed with pump users, but the principles can be applied to discussions about any issue.

In the longer term, pump users will have much more experience of managing their pumps in different situations, and as a result are likely to require much less input from health professionals. There is anecdotal evidence that, over time, people might be less exact about carbohydrate-counting, monitor their blood glucose levels less and rarely adjust their basal rate. However, health professionals' recommendations about these aspects of pump use, as discussed in this chapter, are unlikely to result in behavioural change. Instead, the focus should be kept on the individual pump user: what are they doing, what is working for them, how do they know it is working, what are their main concerns, what are they finding difficult and how could they change the situation to be better for them? These and other questions should form the basis of discussions about their own pump management.

## GROUP EDUCATION FOR INSULIN PUMP USERS

An additional organisational aspect to consider is whether group education can be used for insulin pump therapy. With the national recognition of the benefits of group education (Department of Health, 2005), including being able to share experiences with other people with diabetes and learn from each other, many diabetes teams are looking at ways to integrate group education into more aspects of their diabetes service.

Group education is often used in situations where similar information is required for large numbers of people. Those newly diagnosed with Type 2 diabetes, and people with Type 2 diabetes starting to be treated with insulin are examples of this. However, it should not simply be seen as a time-saving method, as ample evidence exists to demonstrate that educating people in groups provides them with the opportunity to learn from the experiences of others as well as their own. The group process itself is a far more stimulating learning environment than a one-to-one consultation and also engenders a sense of belonging and cohesion rather than of isolation (Elwyn *et al.*, 2004).

To use group education when initiating pump therapy, each session needs to have specific learning outcomes and provide opportunities for pump users to share experiences and develop their problem-solving skills. There are a number of techniques that work well when providing group education sessions, using the philosophy discussed earlier in this chapter, as described in Table 8.3.

For insulin pump services that are just being developed, there might be very small numbers of people to be initiated with a pump and so one-to-one consultations could be the only choice. However, as the service expands and more

**Table 8.3** Techniques to use in group education

| Technique | Examples |
| --- | --- |
| Use a questioning approach to elicit group knowledge. | What do you already know about insulin pump therapy? Why do you think it will be helpful for you? |
| Create an environment where everyone can contribute equally. | Ask people to discuss questions in pairs or small groups before a larger group discussion. Use Post-its or flip charts to gather information. |
| Use a non-judgemental approach to discussion. | Thank people for their contributions. Treat all answers equally. Do not use praise or disapproval. |
| Involve everyone's views. | When answers are suggested, ask for opinions from other group members on the same topic. Facilitate discussions rather than answer direct questions. |
| Use a non-didactic approach to information-giving. | Ask people to identify their main questions or concerns. Develop materials and exercises for group members to work out the answers for themselves. |
| Help people to develop their own problem-solving skills. | Ask people to provide examples of what situations they have found difficult to manage, or situations they believe will be difficult to manage, and involve others in finding solutions. |

people start to use pumps, group education will become possible. Follow-up in groups is useful, in both the short and long term, as this allows people to share experiences and learn from each other. While individual consultations will always have a place in diabetes care, they are unlikely to provide the richness and opportunities for learning that take place in a group education situation, as reflected by the experiences of pump users in Chapter Three.

## CONCLUSION

This chapter has discussed the aims of educating people with diabetes to be able to successfully self-manage their diabetes using insulin pump therapy. It has provided information about an approach that focuses on the needs and wishes of the pump user rather than the traditional approach of focusing on issues the health professional believes are important. It has also provided a number of examples of how this might be put into practice. Group education has also been discussed, including techniques that will facilitate reflection and the development of problem-solving skills. In summary, using the approach outlined in this chapter, the health professional becomes responsible for the process they use during a consultation or group education session, but the content of the discussion is much more directed by the person with diabetes, in this case a pump user.

Educational approaches to diabetes care have long been debated, largely due to the difficulties of describing and replicating interventions and also because health professionals are trained in, and more familiar with, approaches designed for use in acute care situations. To provide more effective education, as described here, information about using a different approach might not be enough, and many documents recommend that health professionals seek out training in this type of approach.

# REFERENCES

Anderson RM, Funnell MM, Butler PM *et al.* (1995) Patient empowerment: Results of a randomized controlled trial. *Diabetes Care* **18**(7): 943–949.

Department of Health (2001) *National Service Framework for Diabetes: Standards*, DH, London.

Department of Health (2005) *Structured Patient Education in Diabetes*, DH, London.

Elwyn G, Greenhalgh T, Macfarlane F (2004) *Groups: A Guide to Small Group Work in Healthcare, Management, Education and Research*, Radcliffe Medical Press, Abingdon.

Evans JMM, Newton RW, Ruta DA *et al.* (1999) Frequency of blood glucose monitoring in relation to glycaemic control: Observational study with diabetes database. *British Medical Journal* **319**(7202): 83–86.

Funnell MM, Anderson RM, Arnold MS *et al.* (1991) Empowerment: An idea whose time has come in diabetes education. *Diabetes Educator* **17**(1): 37–41.

Knight KM, Dornan T, Bundy C (2006) The diabetes educator: Trying hard, but must concentrate more on behaviour. *Diabetic Medicine* **23**(5): 485–501.

Lorig K, Gonzalez V (1992) The integration of theory and practice: A 12-year case study. *Health Education Quarterly* **19**(3): 355–368.

McCann S, Weinman M (1996) Encouraging patient participation in general practice consultations: Effect on consultation length and content, patient satisfaction and health. *Psychology & Health* **11**: 857–869.

Morris AD, Boyle DI, McMahon AD *et al.* (1997) Adherence to insulin treatment, glycaemic control and ketoacidosis in insulin-dependent diabetes mellitus. *The Lancet* **350**(9090): 1505–1510.

National Institute for Health and Clinical Excellence (2003) *Guidance on the use of patient-education models for diabetes*, NICE, London.

Toobert DJ, Hampson SE, Glasgow RE (2000) The summary of diabetes self-care activities measure: Results from 7 studies and a revised scale. *Diabetes Care* **23**(7): 943–950.

Williams G, Freedman ZR, Deci EL (1998) Supporting autonomy to motivate patients with diabetes for glucose control. *Diabetes Care* **21**(10): 1644–1651.

# Chapter 9
# Initiating Insulin Pump Therapy

When someone is starting to use a pump for the first time, a huge amount of information is discussed within a relatively short space of time. Chapter Eight discusses an approach that it can be helpful to adopt, and this chapter provides the practical and technical aspects of starting to use a pump. A step-by-step guide to setting up and programming a pump is included, followed by the type of information that should be included in an initial education programme. Finally, how a training plan could be developed is discussed, with an example of what this might look like.

## STARTING TO USE AN INSULIN PUMP

The information in this section is generic, as the way that different functions are carried out will vary from one type of pump to another, and it is important that the handbooks for each individual pump be closely followed. It can be useful for a potential pump user to first look at a pump that is already set up, for example one filled with saline, to see how some of the functions work before setting it up themselves for the first time. The following sections give a breakdown of the practical aspects of starting to use a pump for the first time.

## Inserting the batteries

Inserting the batteries is the first step. Some insulin pumps have custom-built batteries specific only to that pump, which are obtained directly from the pump manufacturer. However, the majority of pumps now use batteries that can be purchased in shops. If the pump specifies a particular type of battery, such as lithium or alkaline, that indicates which type of battery will offer optimal use and performance. It might be possible to use a different type of battery if the literature accompanying the pump indicates this, but they are likely to have a shorter life and need replacing more often than the recommended batteries. The pumps retain their settings when the batteries are removed for a short period, for example when replacing them. It is important to change the battery as soon as the pump indicates it is getting low rather than waiting for the battery to expire, as the latter can cause the pump to fail.

## Setting the date and time

It is important to set the clock on the pump to the correct time, so that any variation in the basal rate during the day and night is correctly timed. Some pumps provide reminders to set the date and time when the pump is first used or when the battery has been removed for a period of days or weeks. Setting the date will ensure that information stored in the pump's memory will provide an accurate reflection of the insulin doses given. Most pumps offer the option of using a 12-hour or 24-hour clock. The clocks do not automatically adjust for the start and finish of British summertime but have to be altered manually, as they do when travelling across time zones (see Chapter 12).

## The button-pressing sequence

All the currently available insulin pumps have between four and five operating buttons. These buttons are pressed in different sequences to carry out different pump functions. Becoming familiar with these sequences and functions takes time, but a good starting point is to help a pump user understand what 'logic' the pump has to its sequences. This will help them become aware of how to find different menus, which buttons can be used to scroll through options and which buttons select or alter settings. Most pump users initially learn only those functions that they use on a daily basis and take longer to be able to recall how to use less common functions, but being aware of the sequences to go through can make it easier to find less commonly used functions.

## Inserting the insulin reservoir

The next step is to insert the insulin reservoir. If the pump does not take pre-filled insulin cartridges, insulin will need to be drawn up into the reservoir according to the manufacturer's instructions – the size of the reservoir varies between pumps from 1.76 ml (millilitres) up to 3 ml, and with some pumps the pump user has a choice of whether to use a larger or smaller reservoir, depending on their anticipated insulin use. It is generally possible to prepare a number of reservoirs in advance, which can then be stored in the refrigerator until needed. The piston rod needs to be retracted in order to insert the reservoir, which is achieved by pressing the pump buttons in a specific sequence.

## Choosing an infusion set

The different types of infusion sets available for each pump have been described in Chapter Four, and pump users should have the opportunity to try using different types before choosing which they prefer in the longer term. Ease of use for the individual and personal preference are the most important factors in choosing an infusion set. The choice of the initial set needs to be made in the setting-up phase of pump use or during the pre-pump preparation discussions, as the tubing needs to be primed with insulin before being attached to the pump user.

## Priming the pump

Each pump has a priming function, where a set amount of insulin is infused through the tubing. Some pumps can be programmed by the pump user to set specific amounts of insulin needed for priming, while others deliver enough insulin to fill the longest tubing. Careful priming, following the instructions for the individual pump, ensures that no air bubbles are in the tubing. While small amounts of air will cause no harm in themselves if accidentally infused, it means that the insulin dose for that period is not being infused, which can cause hyperglycaemia. Holding the tubing (and adapter for some models of pump) in such a way that the insulin – and air – will rise vertically will help to minimise the likelihood of air bubbles in the tubing. Using insulin at room temperature, rather than straight from the refrigerator, also helps. Priming is complete when a small bead of insulin can be seen at the end of the tubing and no air bubbles are caught in the tubing.

## Starting and stopping the pump

Starting and stopping the pump is often one of the first functions taught to a pump user. Becoming familiar with this function helps the pump user gain confidence and be able to find different menus easily, as well as being able to stop the pump quickly at any time.

## Setting the basal rate

The initial basal rate needs to be programmed for the whole 24-hour period according to the starting dose of insulin agreed (see Chapter 10 for how this is calculated). A flat basal rate is most commonly used to start with, which means that the same amount of insulin is infused every hour. There might be exceptions to this, for example if someone is concerned about nocturnal hypoglycaemia they might want to start with a reduced basal rate overnight. It is useful to keep a written record of the starting basal rates and alterations made, which can be referred to if the pump user accidentally alters the rate and wishes to return to the original rate.

## Setting and giving boluses

Learning about how bolus doses of insulin can be given before attaching the pump to the person using it allows time for experimenting and helps ensure that unwanted boluses aren't given accidentally. Setting different amounts of insulin to give and also the different methods of giving boluses (for example giving the insulin immediately or over a longer time frame) are the most frequently used functions for any pump user, and ones they need to be confident with from the outset. Learning how to cancel boluses that have been programmed in is also useful. More information on the types and use of different boluses can be found in Chapter 10.

## Skin preparation and infusion site choice

Once the above steps are complete, the skin should be prepared for insertion of the cannula or needle. Unless the pump user finds themselves to be particularly prone to infections, there is no need to use antiseptic lotions to cleanse the skin. The area should be dry and clean, and hands washed prior to handling the infusion set. Information on siting the infusion set, maintaining good hygiene and avoiding infusion site infections can be found in Chapter 12.

## Where to wear the pump

A number of different accessory clips and pouches in various colours and materials are available for the pumps, which can be worn on belts, in pockets, clipped to a bra or on arm or leg straps. Some pump users prefer to keep their pump out of sight and so are likely to choose a more discreet pump holder, while others are happy to display their pumps. The pumps are usually supplied with a small number of basic pouches, and additional pouches can be purchased directly from the pump manufacturer by the pump user. Pouches are also available from other sources, for example those listed in the Appendix.

## ADDITIONAL PUMP FUNCTIONS

As well as being able to set up and start to use the pump, the pump user should also be made aware of the other pump functions that they might wish to use. Some of these might be used immediately, while other functions can be left until they have gained more confidence in handling the pump and adjusting insulin doses.

## Using the keylock

Pump users have the option of locking the buttons on the pump, as discussed in Chapter Four, and the keylock is then deactivated temporarily when any type of programming is required. Many pump users feel reassured that this eliminates the possibility of insulin being given by accident, and it can be particularly reassuring for parents of young children. If someone wishes to use this feature, they need to become familiar with how to programme it so that they can remember how to unlock their pump when necessary.

## Accessing the pump memory

The pump user should be taught how to access the pump memory, which is a valuable tool to be able to check what they have programmed into the pump. It also helps them to proactively manage their pump by identifying what variations in insulin doses have been delivered, which can be compared with what glycaemic control has been achieved in different situations.

## Alarm functions

Each pump has a number of different alarms, as discussed in Chapter Four. Learning which alarms require urgent attention and also customising the alarm system where possible to suit the individual pump user will help them make best use of the alarm feature, and also any alarms that have been activated will be stored in the pump's memory and can be accessed again at a later time.

## Altering the basal rate

The pump user is unlikely to need to alter the basal rate on day one, but it is an essential part of early pump management and should be taught from the outset. Identifying how to programme the basal rate and how to ensure the information is retained in the pump will help pump users to become familiar with this function.

## Using the temporary basal rate

The temporary basal rate is a method of increasing or decreasing the amount of basal or continuous insulin that is being infused for a short period. As an example, if someone is unwell, their insulin requirements are likely to increase, and using a temporary increase in the basal rate is a proactive way of preventing hyperglycaemia occurring. For a reduction in the rate, the minimum rate that a pump can deliver is 10 per cent of the programmed basal rate per hour. If the rate needs to be increased, the maximum amount of insulin that can be delivered using the temporary basal rate is 200 per cent per hour, which is double the original programmed rate. More information on how and when to use the temporary basal rate can be found in Chapter 10.

## LEARNING HOW TO MANAGE PUMP THERAPY

While being able to programme and use the pump is important, applying that knowledge to day-to-day situations means the pump user can then optimise the management of their diabetes. How to manage the different pump functions in order to gain optimal benefit from the pump in different situations will not be discussed here, but Table 9.1 lists the important aspects of day-to-day pump management that should be discussed with a new pump user and highlights which chapter of this book provides that information.

An insulin pump offers a variety of options regarding how specific situations can be managed. When someone starts to use a pump, time spent discussing diabetes management offers the opportunity for reviewing their existing knowledge. Also, as discussed in Chapter Eight, their previous experience can be used to identify how different situations can be managed using an insulin pump. How and when to discuss the different aspects shown in

**Table 9.1**　Optimising diabetes management using a pump

| Aspect of pump management | Relevant book section |
|---|---|
| Matching insulin to carbohydrate intake | Chapter 7 |
| Accounting for alcohol | Chapter 7 |
| Setting and adjusting bolus and basal rates | Chapter 10 |
| Treating and avoiding hypoglycaemia | Chapter 11 |
| Treating and avoiding hyperglycaemia | Chapter 11 |
| Frequency of changing infusion sets and sites | Chapter 12 |
| Managing day-to-day situations (physical activity, sexual activity, holidays) | Chapter 12 |
| Discontinuing insulin pump therapy | Chapter 12 |
| Managing illness and admission to hospital | Chapter 15 |

Table 9.1 will be explored later in this chapter. There are also a number of considerations specific to starting to use a pump that need to be discussed with the pump user, as highlighted in the remainder of this section.

## Agreeing blood glucose level targets

Finding out what blood glucose levels someone with diabetes wants to achieve should be discussed prior to the pump being started, and negotiated with them. Someone who has experienced regular severe hypoglycaemia might want to keep their blood glucose levels higher, while someone who is more concerned about the risk of developing long-term complications might want to aim for much tighter blood glucose control. Gaining agreement between the specialist diabetes team and the pump user will ensure realistic expectations for all concerned.

Tightening control very quickly can cause an initial worsening of any complications, particularly retinopathy, so gradual improvements in blood glucose levels, over a few weeks or months, are recommended. It might be wise to initially agree blood glucose levels that are a small improvement on previous readings and then revise this over the first few weeks until a more ideal range has been reached. Chapter 11 provides more information on how to negotiate and agree target blood glucose levels.

## Reducing insulin doses prior to starting a pump

Ideally, when someone inserts a needle or cannula and attaches their insulin-filled pump for the first time, they should have only a small amount of residual insulin in their system. This is to prevent their receiving insulin through the pump at the same time as previously injected insulin is still working, which can increase the chances of hypoglycaemia occurring. The most recent long-acting insulin dose should be reduced and in some cases omitted completely. If a long-acting insulin analogue is being taken, the dose is likely to need to be reduced more than if an isophane insulin is being taken prior to pump therapy, as it will have a longer-lasting effect on blood glucose levels. Any short-term hyperglycaemia that occurs as a result of the reduced longer-acting insulin can be corrected with additional bolus doses once the pump has been connected. Table 9.2 provides a guide on how to reduce long-acting insulin doses prior to using a pump.

Whether the most recent short-acting insulin needs to be altered depends on the type of insulin and also the time lapse between the last injection and the time of connecting the pump. If a rapid-acting analogue insulin is being

**Table 9.2**   How to reduce long-acting insulin doses prior to initiating pump therapy

| Insulin type and frequency | Time of day the pump will be connected | Adjustment to the dose in the 24 hours prior to connecting the pump |
|---|---|---|
| Once daily isophane taken in the morning | Mid/late morning | Omit the morning dose |
|  | Afternoon | Take 50% of the usual morning dose |
| Once daily long-acting analogue taken in the morning | Mid/late morning *or* afternoon | Omit the morning dose |
| Once daily isophane taken at bedtime | Mid/late morning | Take 50% of the usual dose the previous evening |
|  | Afternoon | Take the normal dose the evening before, or it can be reduced by 25% if hypoglycaemia is a major concern |
| Once daily long-acting analogue taken at bedtime | Mid/late morning *or* afternoon | Take 50% of the usual dose the previous evening |
| Twice daily isophane | Mid/late morning | Take 50% of the usual dose the previous evening, omit the morning dose |
|  | Afternoon | Take the usual dose the previous evening, and 50% of the usual morning dose |
| Twice daily long-acting analogue | Mid/late morning *or* afternoon | Take 50% of the usual dose the previous evening, omit the morning dose |

used, the morning dose can be taken as normal as long as there is at least a two-hour gap between that dose and starting the pump. If the time span is shorter, giving only 50 per cent of the dose is recommended, or the dose could be omitted completely. For soluble insulin, any doses given within the five hours prior to the pump being connected should be reduced by 50 per cent.

If someone has forgotten to reduce their insulin prior to starting the pump, particularly their longer-acting insulin, they will need a reduced dose of insulin via their pump until the insulin action from their injection has reduced. This can be done by using a temporary basal rate of around 50 per cent, and also giving less insulin for meal boluses, for the first 12 to 24 hours, depending on the type of longer-acting insulin.

## Contact details for health professionals

While it can be argued that anyone with diabetes should have access to specialist help when they need it, additional support is likely to be needed in the early days of insulin pump therapy, and is viewed by pump users as an extremely important aspect. A new pump user will have been presented with a large amount of new information in a relatively short space of time and will be dealing with both the technology and also how to manage their diabetes differently. In Chapter Three, pump users highlight how important support can be in the early days of using a pump. In addition, in most specialist diabetes teams there is a small core of health professionals who have developed more knowledge and experience with pumps than other team members, and the pump user should have access to this core team. Providing clear contact details and explaining how the system works (for example whether the caller will connect to an answer phone and how soon they will be contacted back) will help to manage people's expectations and provide reassurance that they can access help if required.

## Day-to-day supplies

Ensuring that essential supplies are available is a key aspect of managing insulin pump therapy. Because the pump user is only taking a short-acting insulin, which in most cases is a rapid-acting insulin analogue, any interruption to their supply of insulin for more than two hours is likely to result in a sharp rise in their blood glucose level, with ketoacidosis developing possibly within four to five hours (Attia *et al.*, 1998). Having access to spare insulin, and a means of injecting that insulin, is therefore crucial. The supplies that a pump user should have available at all times are outlined in Chapter 12.

## Obtaining supplies

Disposable supplies for insulin pumps, such as infusion sets and insulin reservoirs, are collectively known as 'consumables'. It is important that pump users are made aware of how they can order supplies and also to reinforce that they should keep at least one week's supplies in hand rather than risk running out of consumables.

## Agreement with the pump user

As previously discussed, when someone is starting to use a pump, the benefits that will be gained (for example reduced frequency of hypoglycaemia or a lower HbA1c level) will have been clearly identified. Some diabetes teams develop written agreements with pump users regarding what measures will be used to denote the success – or failure – of insulin pump therapy. In other areas, these issues are discussed verbally and are likely to be documented by the health professional. Anecdotally, experienced pump centres report that once someone is using an insulin pump, even though they might not meet previously agreed criteria, they will be extremely reluctant to revert to injection therapy. It is therefore important that the diabetes team decide whether written agreements would be helpful. If they decide to follow this route, ideas of what the agreement might contain are shown in Table 9.3.

**Table 9.3**  Ideas for the content of a written agreement between the pump user and the diabetes team

- criteria to determine the success of insulin pump therapy for that individual
- criteria to measure whether insulin pump therapy has been considered unsuccessful and should be discontinued
- responsibilities of the pump user in managing their pump
- how frequently contact is expected with the diabetes team

## DEVELOPING A TRAINING PLAN

Chapter Five provides information about involving the whole of the specialist team in developing an insulin pump service. Planning how insulin pump initiation is going to be managed, including a common core of advice and information, should also involve the whole team to ensure continuity of care and help the education programme meet the criteria of a structured education programme (Department of Health, 2005).

Opinions vary regarding how much education should be provided prior to someone starting to use a pump, how much should be provided on day one of pump therapy and how much should be left until after day one. It is well recognised that large amounts of information given at one time are unlikely to be remembered, and there is commonly a lack of agreement between people with diabetes and health professionals about what has been discussed in consultations (Parkin and Skinner, 2003). It is therefore important that information is focused on the potential pump user's needs at the time, and that the temptation to tell them everything the health professional knows is avoided. On the other hand, it is also important that the health professional does not prejudge how much someone with diabetes is able to absorb and withhold information unnecessarily. Getting the balance right can be tricky, which is why agreement within the specialist team, and a consistent approach, will help. The following sections provide some suggestions and guidance regarding how an insulin pump education programme could be structured, and an example of a plan is also included in Table 9.4. Much of the education required can be provided in a group setting, which is discussed in Chapter Eight. Planning ahead will help to ensure that any health professionals involved will have the time available to provide a comprehensive programme, as appointments can be booked in advance.

## Before initiating pump therapy

During the assessment phase, when discussions are being held regarding whether insulin pump therapy is a suitable treatment option for an individual, many diabetes teams recommend that the potential pump user attend a structured education programme for people with Type 1 diabetes, if they have not done so already. This helps them to learn (or refresh their previous learning) about assessing their carbohydrate intake and adjusting their mealtime insulin doses according to what they are eating. Gaining confidence in carbohydrate assessment and related insulin adjustment prior to using a pump means the pump user has less to learn at the outset of changing to a pump. It can also result in some people with diabetes deciding that they do not wish to proceed to using a pump, as they are able to manage their diabetes more successfully simply through more proactive management of their insulin doses.

Following the Type 1 education course, the diabetes team need agreement regarding how quickly individuals can move to pump therapy. Giving people time to try out their new method of insulin adjustment can take a few months, or there might be situations where it seems appropriate to initiate pump therapy within a shorter timescale, so identifying what those situations might be will help a consistent approach to be developed.

**Table 9.4** Example of an initial training plan

| Stage of training | Action to be taken |
|---|---|
| Following an initial assessment | Attend the local Type 1 education programme if not already doing so |
| Six months later: one-hour appointment | Assess glycaemic control and improvements following education programme<br>Discuss carbohydrate assessment and insulin adjustment<br>Discuss if a pump is still needed and wanted<br>If yes, demonstrate different pumps and decide which one the person wants to use<br>Put in touch with established pump users<br>Agree a training date |
| No more than two weeks prior to initiating pump therapy: one- to two-hour appointment | Practise handling the pump and using different functions, and try out different cannulae/needles<br>Discuss expectations and lifestyle needs<br>Prepare for day one: what supplies are needed, insulin doses just before starting the pump, basal and bolus rates<br>Wear the pump with saline in for 24–48 hours |
| Pump start day: six- to seven-hour appointment | Set the pump up with insulin, check or programme basal rates<br>Agree insulin to carbohydrate ratios for the pump<br>Check ability to carry out basic pump functions<br>Assess blood glucose levels during pump use over the duration of the appointment<br>Plan the frequency of blood glucose tests and initial targets to aim for<br>Agree action to take if blood glucose levels are outside the initial target range<br>Plan overnight management of the pump<br>Plan insulin dose changes for varying activities over the next two days |
| Two days later: one- to two-hour appointment | Review records in detail, check insulin doses, carbohydrate assessment, management of different situations<br>Make changes to infusion rates if necessary<br>Practise changing the insulin reservoir, priming and changing the cannula or needle |
| Ongoing early follow-up: appointments as required (no less than weekly for the first three weeks) | Review records as above<br>Revise blood glucose targets as required<br>Discuss and encourage proactive management of different situations |

If someone chooses to go ahead with starting to use a pump, the following are most likely to be useful *prior* to the day of initiation:

- Having opportunities to talk to at least one established pump user, or ideally two or three people using pumps.
- Being able to handle a pump, practise setting it up and pressing buttons to carry out different functions.
- Wearing the pump attached to them (infusing saline) for at least 24 hours, or possibly a few days.
- Discussing their lifestyle and what specific aspects will require alterations to their insulin doses using a pump.
- Calculating their initial basal rate and their insulin bolus ratios in relation to both carbohydrate intake and to treating high blood glucose levels.
- Agreeing what blood glucose levels are going to be aimed for initially and what the longer-term aims will be.
- Ensuring that adequate supplies of insulin (rapid-acting for the pump, long-acting to have in reserve), blood glucose testing strips and a method for testing for ketones have been obtained.
- Agreeing what insulin doses should be taken in the 24 hours prior to starting to use the pump.
- Discussing expectations of the pump, agreeing targets and criteria for measuring the success of insulin pump therapy.
- Discuss (and demonstrate/practise) the range of pump functions.
- Look at needles and cannulae, try them out and decide which is preferred.

Ideally, all the above should take place, or as a minimum be revisited, no more than two weeks prior to the pump start; otherwise, it will be more difficult for the individual to remember the pump functions and management strategies.

## On the day of the pump start

The main aim of this appointment is to ensure that the pump user can *safely* manage their insulin pump until their next review, which should be within two to three days of starting to use a pump. By the time they leave the appointment after starting to use a pump, they need to be confident in only a small number of areas of pump management. These include:

- switching the pump on and off
- calculating bolus doses in relation to their carbohydrate intake and to correct hyperglycaemia
- giving bolus doses of insulin

- changing the basal rate
- how to treat hypoglycaemia
- how to resite the cannula or needle
- what to do if they have problems or an emergency situation
- developing a plan of how frequently they will be testing their blood glucose levels, what levels to aim for and what action to take for readings outside their ideal range
- developing a plan for any activities over the next few days (e.g. dining with friends or undertaking physical activity).

During the appointment, the pump user should be able to fill the insulin reservoir, set up the pump, prime the tubing, insert the cannula or needle, set (or check) basal infusion rates and confidently programme boluses into their pump.

Many people first starting to use a pump are naturally cautious and prefer to disrupt their usual routine, for example missing their regular workouts in the gym, in order to try and establish their basal insulin requirements and avoid situations that will adversely affect their glycaemic control. Others prefer to try and manage their normal daily activities using their insulin pump rather than change their routine. Using a questioning approach, as outlined in Chapter Eight, will help to determine how much someone understands about managing a situation and also what they are likely to do when that situation occurs. Management plans should be seen as experimental, as it is important not to instil a sense of failure if the initial plans don't work. Pump users should not be made to feel they have to get perfect results immediately, or see it as a test of their skill in managing their diabetes. Helping the individual develop their own safety guidelines, including what higher or lower levels of blood glucose would prompt them to take action, is a more helpful approach. Also, identifying any key areas that are causing them anxiety, and working with them to find solutions, will help their confidence.

Before they leave on day one, it is also important to discuss and agree on how frequently they will be testing their blood glucose levels, that they understand how to interpret their results in relation to the timing of their meals and bolus doses of insulin and what action to take on the results.

## At the first follow-up appointment

This appointment is primarily to review the pump user's experiences so far, identifying successful and less successful management strategies, refresh knowledge and look at what the pump user now needs to do. Assessing glycaemic control is discussed in Chapter 11, including what record-keeping can be helpful. Asking them to identify what worked and what didn't work for them provides a useful insight, before looking in detail at each part of each day (what blood glucose levels were, what food was eaten, what insulin was delivered and any other factors that were affecting their blood glucose levels at that time). The aim is for the pump user to gain confidence and competence in their decision-making, so encouraging them to suggest what changes might be needed to basal rates or bolus doses will help towards this goal.

Practical skills should also be reviewed: the pump user might already have changed their cannula or needle, but, if not, this might be something they feel apprehensive about, and being able to practise changing the infusion site at this appointment is useful. Filling the insulin reservoir and priming the infusion set are aspects that the majority of pump users don't need to do on a daily basis, and it can be helpful to offer them the opportunity to revisit these skills at this appointment. If new experiences or activities are to be undertaken, creating a management plan in advance, as discussed earlier, will increase their chances of success.

## Ongoing follow-up

After the first follow-up appointment, timescales can vary regarding how frequently people need, or wish, to be seen. Agreeing individual follow-up plans is important at this stage. Some people might have significant events happening in the near future that require variations to the programming of their pump, and they might wish to have regular contact with the health professional. Others might want to experiment on their own, for example they might want to try adjusting their basal rates before they come back for review. While account should be taken of people's different preferences, appointments that are too infrequent at this stage – for example more than a week apart – can result in the individual managing their pump less proactively. Some people prefer to tread cautiously and won't initially make basal rate changes except through discussion when they return for review, so less frequent appointments can mean that it takes much longer to gain satisfactory glycaemic control. With experience, it is possible to identify what scale of follow-up appointments works best within a specialist team to achieve optimum results.

## CONCLUSION

This chapter has provided a step-by-step guide to the technical and practical aspects of starting to use a pump, including a guide to the areas of clinical management that need to be addressed, with signposting to other areas of this book for more information. It has provided guidance on how to develop an initial training plan, and ongoing follow-up and support are discussed in Chapter Five. It can be daunting when starting to use insulin pump therapy within a specialist diabetes team, but careful planning ahead of time regarding how the initiation of therapy will be carried out will help to ensure that a comprehensive and useful training package is delivered.

## REFERENCES

Attia N, Jones T, Holcombe J, Tamborlane W (1998) Comparison of human regular and lispro insulins after interruption of continuous subcutaneous insulin infusion and in the treatment of acutely decompensated IDDM. *Diabetes Care* **21**(5): 817–820.

Department of Health (2005) *Structured Patient Education in Diabetes*, DH, London.

Parkin T, Skinner TC (2003) Discrepancies between patient and professionals recall and perception of an outpatient consultation. *Diabetic Medicine* **20**(11): 909–914.

# Chapter 10
# Setting and Adjusting Insulin Doses

This chapter focuses specifically on setting and adjusting basal and bolus rates of insulin, as this is a key part of successfully managing insulin pump therapy. First, the chapter will look at basal rates: how to set the infusion rate when starting to use insulin pump therapy and how to adjust it on an ongoing basis. Temporary basal rates will then be discussed, with information on how to use them and in what circumstances. Following this, the remainder of the chapter will focus on bolus doses, highlighting the different types of boluses and their meaning, how to calculate food boluses and the use of correction boluses to deal with hyperglycaemia.

## SETTING AN INITIAL BASAL RATE

The term 'basal rate' refers to the amount of insulin that is delivered continuously by the pump over a 24-hour period, to meet the body's need for a continuous supply of insulin. It is programmed in advance and is then delivered automatically without the need for additional button-pressing by the pump user.

Before an individual starts to wear a pump, the amount of insulin that is going to be delivered via the basal rate needs to be decided. There is no robust evidence to support one method of calculation over another. Body weight can be used as a guide, but this is likely to overestimate an individual's needs; using pre-pump insulin doses as a starting point is likely to be more realistic, even though the individual might not have had good glycaemic control previously. It is also important to use doses cautiously to avoid hypoglycaemia. In the longer term, the basal rate can be closely tailored to meet each pump user's needs.

Some experienced specialist teams have developed their own algorithms regarding what basal rates to use as a starting point, based on the pump user's previous injected insulin doses. None of these has been subjected to rigorous

**Table 10.1**  Examples of calculations of initial basal rates

| Total daily pre-pump insulin dose | 28 units | 45 units | 60 units |
|---|---|---|---|
| Reduce by 30% | 30% = 8 | 30% = 13 | 30% = 18 |
| | New dose = 20 | New dose = 32 | New dose = 42 |
| Divide by 2 | = 10 | = 16 | = 21 |
| Divide by 24 | = 0.4 | = 0.6 | = 0.8 |
| Hourly infusion rate: | 0.4 units | 0.6 units | 0.8 units |

trials, although that is also true of the many different ways commonly used to adjust injected doses of insulin. A standard insulin decrease can be used, as follows:

1. Take the total pre-pump daily dose of injected insulin prior to starting pump therapy.
2. Reduce this by 30 per cent.
3. Divide the remaining total by 2.
4. Divide the new total by 24 to give a flat hourly infusion rate.

Examples of how this works in practice are seen in Table 10.1. It will be seen from the example that where it is difficult to calculate the dose exactly the number in each case has been rounded *down*, rather than up, to reduce the potential for hypoglycaemia to occur. Once a specialist team becomes more experienced, they can develop their own algorithm that they prefer to use, which might be different from the example quoted.

There can be times when the calculations might be varied for particular individual circumstances. For example, if someone has very frequent hypoglycaemia, the total daily insulin dose might be reduced by more than 30 per cent. Similarly, if someone rarely experiences hypoglycaemia but instead has continual high blood glucose readings before starting pump therapy, a smaller reduction in the total daily insulin dose might be needed. However it is calculated, it is highly unlikely that the initial basal rate will match the individual's exact requirements; instead, it should be considered a starting point only, from which adjustments can be made to optimise the effect on blood glucose levels.

## ONGOING ADJUSTMENT OF BASAL RATES

When adjusting the basal rate, the most important aspect is to ensure that the changes are made early enough to be effective. For example, if hypoglycaemia is experienced, the basal rate can be changed for the hour when the hypoglycaemia occurs, but the hour prior to that is also likely to need changing. In most circumstances, either increasing or decreasing the basal rate for a two-hour period is likely to be more useful than changing a single hour.

For the first 24 to 48 hours of insulin pump therapy, some residual intermediate or long-acting insulin from the previously used injection therapy might still have an influence over blood glucose levels. Therefore, making precise adjustments to basal rates for long-term use is not possible at this stage. If the pump user is experiencing hypoglycaemia, however, the basal rate (if that appears to be the cause) should be reduced to prevent this happening the next day. As already indicated, it is important to reduce the basal rate early enough to be effective, so the dose should be reduced in the hour when hypoglycaemia has occurred, plus the hour before this, and initially reductions should be made in 0.1 unit increments per hour. If hypoglycaemia still occurs, these two hours can be further reduced, but it also might be necessary to reduce the dose the hour prior to these by 0.1 units.

Once the first few days of pump therapy are over, it is likely that the only insulin having an effect is that being delivered via the pump, and basal rates can start to be assessed and adjusted in detail.

## Assessing and adjusting the basal rate

If the basal rate is set correctly, blood glucose readings before meals, before bed and around two o'clock in the morning are likely to be within the target range (see Chapter 11 for more information on setting individual targets). To assess individual parts of the day or night, readings taken no more than three to four hours apart can indicate whether there is a trend of blood glucose levels rising or falling. It is also possible to miss a meal to be able to assess the basal rate over that time period, which can be particularly helpful in the early stages of using a pump. If a meal is missed, the basal rate should keep blood glucose levels fairly constant during that time.

It is important to assess trends rather than individual readings, so the difference between two readings is likely to be more significant than the readings themselves. Looking at whether the basal rate has risen or fallen from the previous reading, for example, will indicate what adjustments are required. A reading of 9 mmol/l (millimoles per litre) might be considered too high, but if it has fallen from 12 mmol/l two hours ago it has dropped rather than risen, so the basal rate at that point should be decreased rather than increased. As a general rule, if the difference between two readings is 3 mmol/l or more, altering the basal rate is likely to be worthwhile to prevent this happening in the future. Table 10.2 provides examples to illustrate how adjustments to the basal rate can be made.

**Table 10.2**  Examples of how to make adjustments to the basal rate

---

**Example 1:** blood glucose is 12.5 mmol/l at 9 a.m., then falls to 9 mmol/l at 11.30 a.m. *Action:* if the 9 a.m. reading has risen from an earlier reading, increase the basal rate from 7 a.m. to 9 a.m. by 0.1 units per hour. Also, decrease the basal rate from 9 a.m. to 11 a.m. by 0.1 units per hour.

**Example 2:** blood glucose levels are reaching the target range most of the day, but are too high around 4–5 p.m. *Action:* increase the basal rate by 0.1 units per hour from 2 p.m. to 4 p.m. and reassess.

---

If it is difficult to identify what changes are needed, blood glucose readings can be collected over a few days and the trends assessed before altering the basal rate. The exception to assessing trends over a few days is when unexplained night-time hypoglycaemia occurs. In this situation, it is more prudent to change the basal rate immediately and then reassess the effect rather than risk an occurrence of the hypoglycaemia.

Each hour should be adjusted by 0.1 unit only as already discussed, unless the person demonstrates marked insulin resistance, in which case 0.2 units per hour might be used, although this is relatively rare. The only major exception is pregnancy, where larger adjustments might be needed in the third trimester (see Chapter 14 for more information). Once changes have been made to the basal rates, their effect should be assessed using blood glucose readings over the following few days, and further changes should be made if necessary.

Basal rates should be regularly reviewed, as it is easy for a pump user to get into the habit of reactively correcting blood glucose readings, or eating to avoid hypoglycaemia, rather than changing the basal rate. They also should be assessed whenever there is a change of circumstances for the pump user, such as weight gain or loss or if activity levels change. In some circumstances, such as being unwell, insulin requirements can change quite rapidly, whereas in others, such as weight loss or gain, the change is likely to be more gradual and might not easily be noticed. Table 10.3 gives examples of when basal rates are likely to need increasing or decreasing.

The changes that are required for individuals will vary, but pump users might be able to establish their own general pattern. For example, some women will notice a change in their blood glucose levels around the time of menstruation, such as a rise in their readings for a couple of days prior to their period, but others can find that their blood glucose level only increases when their period starts. The effect of stress also varies greatly from one individual to another. Working with each person will help to establish what their own variations in blood glucose levels are and whether those variations are significant enough to need to alter the basal rate.

**Table 10.3** When changes are likely to be required to basal rates

| Basal rates might need increasing: | Basal rates might need decreasing: |
|---|---|
| • if weight increases | • if weight decreases |
| • when infections or illness occur | • when overall physical activity is increased |
| • when overall physical activity is decreased | • if hypoglycaemia starts to occur for no other reason |
| • around the time of menstruation | |
| • following prolonged periods of stress | |
| • when taking steroids | |
| • if frequent hyperglycaemia starts to occur for no other reason | |

## Additional considerations

Insulin sensitivity will vary through the day, so most people are likely to need a variable basal rate. However, it is unlikely that major variations will be needed from one hour to the next, so assessing overall trends in the basal rate is important. For example, if someone has been reducing their basal rate to avoid hypoglycaemia, they might have two consecutive hours with 0.7 units per hour being infused followed immediately by two hours with 0.1 units per hour being infused. Making the reduction in the basal rate earlier will result in a more gradual decrease in the dose, so for example the pump could be programmed to deliver 0.6, 0.5, 0.3 and 0.2 units per hour respectively over the same four-hour period. The same amount of insulin is given, but the new rates ensure that less insulin is delivered at an earlier time and are more likely to prevent hypoglycaemia effectively. Pump users often get into the habit of adjusting their insulin very close to the blood glucose levels they wish to influence, and taking a wider view is usually more productive.

It is possible to set more than one basal rate, either on the pump itself or with the aid of a computer program that stores additional basal rates which can be downloaded as required depending on the changes in the pump user's daily routine. Anecdotally, people rarely use more than half a dozen different basal rates and are most likely to use a single basal rate. Multiple basal rates can be useful when someone works shifts or regularly has days that vary in their level of activity. They can also be used for young children, if they have different activities on different days, to avoid parents needing to reprogramme the pump each week.

In summary, any adjustment of basal rates should be relatively slow and incremental in most instances, and adjusting a lot of different hours without giving enough time to assess the effect can lead to erratic blood glucose control and make it difficult to work out what adjustments are needed. Also, as a general guide, an individual is unlikely to need more than about 60 per cent of their total daily insulin dose as their basal rate.

## TEMPORARY BASAL RATES

A temporary basal rate can be programmed into an insulin pump when either more or less insulin is required over a relatively short time. For example, if someone is undertaking physical activity, their insulin requirements are likely to drop, whereas, if they are unwell, they are likely to experience a rise in blood glucose levels and therefore need more insulin. The temporary basal rate is programmed in at the time it needs to be commenced and is measured as a percentage increase or decrease from the original basal rate. The pump user also needs to select how long the altered basal rate should continue. In general, it takes about an hour for a temporary basal rate to become effective, so, if a change in insulin requirements can be predicted (which might not always be possible), programming an hour before this time will help to keep the blood glucose levels in the target range.

A basal rate decrease can be set to as low as 10 per cent, or up to 90 per cent, which are percentages of the usual hourly rate that is already programmed into the pump. For example, if the temporary basal rate is set at 50 per cent for three hours and the pump was originally programmed to deliver 0.6, 0.4 and 0.2 units respectively in those hours, it will deliver 0.3, 0.2 and 0.1 units instead, before returning to the usual basal rate at the end of the three-hour period. If less insulin is required, for example when undertaking physical activity, it is important to start the temporary basal rate early enough to avoid hypoglycaemia, as previously discussed. (See Chapter 12 for more information on managing physical activity.)

Increases in the basal rate can be set from 110 per cent to 200 per cent, so a maximum of double the usual basal rate can be given if necessary. If a pump user finds they are administering a number of correction doses to deal with hyperglycaemia resulting from illness or other causes, using a temporary basal rate increase will prevent their blood glucose rising as high, and potentially mean they have less need to give additional correction doses. Chapter 15 contains more information on dealing with illness.

It is important to remember that the pump user can cancel a temporary basal rate at any time if they feel it is no longer required, such as when a sports session is cancelled, so they can immediately revert back to their usual basal rate. Pump users might need encouragement to use the temporary basal rate function, particularly if they have not used it in the early days of pump therapy, and will need help and practice to become confident in its use.

## BOLUS DOSES OF INSULIN

The term 'bolus' refers to an amount of insulin that is programmed by the pump user, in addition to the basal rate, in response to an identified need for insulin at that time. There are two main categories: food boluses (sometimes referred to as 'meal boluses'), to match carbohydrate intake, and correction boluses, to manage high blood glucose levels. Each pump user will develop their own ratios of how much insulin they need to keep their blood glucose within, or close to, their target range. While equations to calculate bolus doses often appear relatively straightforward, many people find it difficult to work out percentages, divisions and multiplications. Part of the education package offered should include helping them have a clear understanding of how they can calculate the amount of insulin they need.

## Types of bolus that pumps can deliver

As well as determining the amount of insulin needed, pump users have a choice of how they want their bolus to be delivered. The total dose required can be given immediately or extended over a longer timescale. Table 10.4 provides information about the types of boluses that pumps can deliver. Also, different terms are used by different pump manufacturers, and the table shows the terms that might be used as well as providing the generic terms used throughout this book.

## FOOD BOLUSES

Chapter Seven describes how to calculate insulin to carbohydrate ratios, usually described as the amount of insulin needed for 10 grams of carbohydrate, or one carbohydrate portion (1 CP). If someone is already adjusting their mealtime doses of insulin according to their food's carbohydrate content prior to

**Table 10.4** Types of boluses that pumps can deliver

| Bolus name | Alternative names | How insulin is delivered |
|---|---|---|
| Standard | Normal | immediately |
| Extended | Square wave | at a constant rate over a specified number of hours |
| Mixed | Multiwave, Dual wave, Combo | part immediately, part at a constant rate over a specified number of hours |

starting to use pump therapy, they can use the same insulin to carbohydrate ratio with their pump and assess its effectiveness with their blood glucose readings. If not, a standard ratio of one unit to 10 grams of carbohydrate can be used as a starting point.

Once someone has calculated the carbohydrate content of their food and decided how much insulin they need, the type of bolus to give needs to be determined, as described in Table 10.4 above. The total amount of carbohydrate in a meal, its Glycaemic Index and the amount of protein and fat it contains will all affect how quickly the food is broken down and therefore indicate how quickly or slowly the insulin is likely to be needed. As a general rule, meals containing more than 50 grams of carbohydrate, or those that are high in fat and protein, are absorbed more slowly and are therefore likely to require insulin to be delivered over a longer period, using an extended or mixed bolus. Research suggests that, in these circumstances, if a mixed bolus is used, the larger part, around 70 per cent of the total bolus, should be delivered immediately and the remaining 30 per cent more slowly (Chase *et al.*, 2002).

An alternative to using the different bolus functions for high-carbohydrate and high-fat/protein meals is to split the total dose and give it in two parts. As when using the mixed bolus option, this is likely to be most effective when 70 per cent of the total dose is given as the initial bolus and 30 per cent as the second bolus. Chapter Seven provides more detail on how to use the different bolus functions in relation to food intake, including the optimal timing of doses.

To assess whether a food bolus is having the desired effect, taking blood glucose readings before a meal and again two hours after the insulin bolus will help pump users to assess the effect of their food bolus. If the amount of insulin is correct, the blood glucose level taken after the meal should have returned to within 2 mmol/l of the pre-meal reading. If a correction bolus (discussed in the next section) has been given before the meal, the effect of that should also be taken into consideration and the blood glucose level should be proportionally lower. For example, if the blood glucose was 10 mmol/l before a meal, a pump user with a correction ratio of one unit to 2.5 mmol might give two units to correct this, which should bring the blood glucose down to 5 mmol, and the aim of the food bolus is to then keep the blood glucose level close to 5 mmol/l.

Once someone has established their insulin to carbohydrate ratio, this should not be changed on the basis of one or two readings. If the ratio does not seem to be effective, pre- and post-meal blood glucose levels should be taken for three days in order to decide what changes to the ratio are needed. Also, any changes to the ratio should be assessed through blood glucose testing to see whether they are effective. Some people find that they need different insulin to carbohydrate ratios at different times of the day, in line with their varied insulin sensitivity, so might use a different ratio for different meals.

## CORRECTION BOLUSES

'Correction bolus' is the term used to describe an additional dose of insulin that is given to bring high blood glucose readings to within the target range, independent of food boluses. Correction boluses can be given at any time of the day or night, although high blood glucose levels less than two hours after eating might simply mean that the food bolus has not yet had its full effect, in which case a correction dose might not be needed.

Most pump users start by using a standard correction ratio of one unit to 2.5 mmol/l. This means that, if insulin is given when no carbohydrate is being eaten, each unit of insulin would be expected to reduce the blood glucose level by 2.5 mmol/l. An alternative method of calculating the correction dose is to use what is known as the '100 rule'. The number 100 is divided by the total daily insulin dose, to give the expected number of millimoles the blood glucose would fall by when one unit of insulin is given. This can be useful as an ongoing reference to assess whether the correction dose used is close to this amount, but it has limited use when first starting to use a pump.

Examples of how correction doses can be calculated, using different correction ratios, are shown in Table 10.5. The pump user should first identify

**Table 10.5**   Examples of insulin correction doses

| Starting blood glucose level (mmol/l) | Target range (mmol/l) | Correction ratio | Amount of insulin given (units) | Blood glucose level two hours later (to one decimal point) (mmol/l) |
|---|---|---|---|---|
| 12.0 | 4–7 | 1 unit to 2.5 mmol/l | 2.0 | 7.0 |
|  |  |  | 2.5 | 5.7 |
| 10.5 | 4–7 | 1 unit to 2.5 mmol/l | 1.5 | 6.7 |
|  |  |  | 2.0 | 5.5 |
| 8.6 | 4–7 | 1 unit to 2.5 mmol/l | 1.0 | 6.1 |
|  |  |  | 1.5 | 4.8 |
| 12.0 | 4–7 | 1 unit to 4 mmol/l | 1.5 | 6.0 |
|  |  |  | 2.0 | 4.0 |
| 10.5 | 4–7 | 1 unit to 4 mmol/l | 1.0 | 6.5 |
|  |  |  | 1.5 | 4.5 |
| 8.6 | 4–7 | 1 unit to 4 mmol/l | 0.5 | 6.6 |
|  |  |  | 1.0 | 4.6 |

what blood glucose level they want to achieve and then calculate how many millimoles per litre drop that entails. From this, they can apply their correction ratio to identify how much insulin they need to give. As the examples show, in some cases more than one choice of correction dose will still bring the blood glucose level within the target range. Initially, pump users might wish to aim for levels at the higher end of their target range but, as they gain confidence that hypoglycaemia isn't likely, will become more confident to aim for tighter glycaemic control. To find out whether the correction ratio is correct, the blood glucose should be checked two hours later and compared with the level that was anticipated.

Calculation charts are produced by the pump manufacturers that can be helpful to be able to work out the amount of insulin which is needed, based on the current blood glucose level, correction ratio and target blood glucose range. Also, as discussed in Chapter Four, some insulin pumps can be programmed with correction ratios and target blood glucose levels, and on that basis can suggest what amount of correction bolus is needed.

Although each pump user will have a correction ratio, if their blood glucose is at a much higher level initially, they are likely to have a greater degree of insulin resistance and so might need a slightly higher correction ratio if their blood glucose is 16 mmol/l, for example, than if they were correcting a blood glucose of 9 mmol/l. Standard correction ratios can be tried as a starting point, and as the pump user becomes more experienced they might find that they require a different ratio if their blood glucose level is higher. Experimentation, and frequent blood glucose testing to monitor the result, will help to determine this.

Correction boluses are necessary whenever the blood glucose rises above the target range. This is likely to occur when unwell and during periods of reduced activity but also can occur at any point, which is why frequent blood glucose monitoring is important. If frequent corrections are required, the basal rate should be reassessed, as the hourly rates might have to be amended to prevent the rises in blood glucose levels. Also, if correction doses are required before meals, ideally they should be given at least 10 minutes before eating, to enable the correction bolus to start taking effect.

There is potential for pump users to give correction doses without either reflecting on the cause or thinking about how it can be prevented in the future. If this happens frequently, it means that the pump user could be spending a significant amount of time with their blood glucose outside the desired range, contributing to a raised HbA1c and poor glycaemic control. Correction doses should therefore be encouraged at an early stage so that they become a normal part of pump management, but also reflecting on what caused the hyperglycaemia will help the pump user to be proactive in preventing a recurrence of the same situation. The management of hyperglycaemia, including what action to take if the blood glucose does not respond to an initial correction dose, is explained in detail in Chapter 11.

## CONCLUSION

This chapter has outlined how to manage basal and bolus doses of insulin when using pump therapy, to optimise glycaemic control. As has been discussed, there are standard ways of assessing this, but there are also many variations that can be applied in different circumstances. Blood glucose testing and accurate record-keeping to identify what causes fluctuations in blood glucose levels are the main tools to be able to accurately assess whether the infusion rates being used are successful. Pump users should be encouraged to experiment and to alter their rates if they feel they need to, as this will help them gain confidence in making changes and will also enable them to take a proactive approach in adapting their existing knowledge about their insulin doses to any new situations they encounter.

## REFERENCE

Chase HP, Saib Z, Mackenzie T *et al.* (2002) Post-prandial glucose excursions following four methods of bolus insulin administration in subjects with Type 1 diabetes. *Diabetic Medicine* **19**(4): 317–321.

Chapter 11
# Optimising Glycaemic Control

Gaining good glycaemic control is one of the main reasons for using insulin pump therapy. Evidence has already been discussed in Chapter One which has demonstrated that pump use can reduce HbA1c levels, reduce the incidence and severity of hypoglycaemia (particularly at night), improve hypoglycaemia awareness, reduce the risk of ketoacidosis and produce less variation in blood glucose levels from day to day. The general principles of how to achieve good glycaemic control with injection therapy, which include analysing trends in blood glucose readings and being proactive rather than simply reactive, still apply to insulin adjustments when using a pump. However, not having to deal with the variable absorption and action of long-acting insulin and having the ability to make very precise changes in insulin doses mean that blood glucose levels close to those of people without diabetes can be achieved more readily.

This chapter will discuss ways of reducing variations and working towards achieving normal blood glucose levels. It will first discuss blood glucose monitoring, including when to monitor and what glycaemic targets to aim for, initially and in the longer term, what records to keep and how blood glucose levels can be reviewed in consultations. It will then discuss the detection, management and prevention of hypoglycaemia and hyperglycaemia.

## BLOOD GLUCOSE MONITORING

Blood glucose monitoring is one of the most useful tools for someone managing their insulin pump therapy and for them to gain good glycaemic control. It is difficult to be prescriptive about how much monitoring will help someone to successfully manage their pump therapy, but there are general principles that can be used as a starting point. It is important to ensure that pump users are not continually reacting to individual readings but instead are assessing trends and taking appropriate action.

# When to monitor

Frequent blood glucose monitoring, especially in the early stages of pump therapy, can help a pump user adjust their basal rates and also their food boluses to closely match their insulin needs. It is important that potential pump users understand how frequently they will need to monitor, both in the early stages and on an ongoing basis.

The minimum recommendations when first using a pump are to monitor blood glucose levels at least eight times a day. These readings should be taken before each meal, two hours after each meal, before going to bed and in the middle of the night (around 2 to 3 a.m.). This provides the pump user with information that can then be used to adjust insulin doses, as shown in Table 11.1. Many pump users like to test more frequently than this when first using a pump, to reassure themselves about their blood glucose levels even if no action is required. It can be a time of high anxiety, as many pump users have used injection therapy for many years, which, even if it did not produce good glycaemic control, was a familiar system to them. Switching to using a pump, and learning how to manage diabetes in a new way, can seem to be as complex as first being diagnosed. It can also seem strange to no longer have to give injections, and blood glucose monitoring results act as reassurance and so build confidence that the pump is delivering the programmed insulin doses.

Over the longer term, it is recommended that pump users monitor their blood glucose at least four times a day, before meals and before bed, which are the main times when decisions need to be made about insulin doses. The downside of only testing this frequently is that the results of dose adjustments, for example insulin given at mealtimes, are not known. Pump users should be

**Table 11.1**  Information gathered from blood glucose testing

| Blood glucose test | What information it provides |
| --- | --- |
| Pre-meals | identifies whether the basal rate is correctly set for the previous few hours and is a starting point to assess whether the meal bolus is correct |
| Two hours after meals | identifies whether the meal bolus is correct: it should be within 2 mmol/l of the pre-meal blood glucose |
| Before going to bed | identifies whether the basal rate is set correctly for the previous few hours and gives the pump user a starting point to make decisions about what to do with the basal rate overnight |
| 2–3 a.m. | provides a midpoint check of what is happening with blood glucose readings during the night, to assess the basal rate in the first and second halves of the night |

encouraged to regularly incorporate some days into their routine when more frequent blood glucose monitoring can be carried out, including middle-of-the-night testing. In practice, pump users often report that they test their blood glucose more frequently than four times a day as a routine, as it helps them make proactive decisions and stay in control of their diabetes.

There are a number of other times when testing will be useful, including:

- when someone has no awareness of hypoglycaemia
- when checking the effect of a food bolus
- before driving
- before and after physical activity
- when unwell
- when alcohol has been consumed
- when insulin doses have been varied (e.g. a temporary basal rate has been used, a correction bolus has been given or the pump has been taken off for a short period)
- when specific individual difficulties (e.g. gastroparesis) make blood glucose levels less predictable
- two hours after changing an infusion set to ensure insulin is being delivered.

The reason for the above tests is to gather information about whether the pump management has been successful, and also to ensure that pump users are not putting themselves at risk. If they are encouraged to think about blood glucose readings in terms of 'information', pump users can more readily identify how much information will be useful to them to manage their insulin pump therapy. It is also important that they have a simple, logical means of documenting their results so that they can review the information collected. More information on documentation of results can be found later in this chapter.

Continuous glucose monitoring can have a place in pump management, for example if erratic patterns of blood glucose levels start to appear with no obvious cause or if hypoglycaemia becomes difficult to manage. Some pump users will choose to use this regularly, although NHS funding is limited and they might have to self-fund this method of monitoring. Discussing the results and the usefulness of this method of testing with them will help them determine how to use it to their best advantage.

Having the means to test ketones is also important, and is discussed later in this chapter and also in Chapter 15. Some pump users use urine testing strips for ketone testing, but it is becoming more common for pump users to have blood glucose meters that can also test for ketones. Most specialist teams will provide these meters when someone is first starting to use an insulin pump.

**Table 11.2** Interpretation of blood glucose results

| Blood glucose readings (mmol/l) | | Interpretation |
|---|---|---|
| 10 a.m.: 10 | 12.30 p.m.: 10.1 | despite the readings being too high, the basal rate is set correctly between these two times |
| 10 a.m.: 10 | 12.30 p.m.: 4.5 | despite the second reading being within the target range, the basal rate is set too high as it has caused a drop of 5.5 mmol/l within two hours |
| Pre-lunch: 9.4 | Two hours post-lunch: 9.8 | assuming no correction dose was given, the lunch bolus is correct |

# Understanding the results

How to adjust insulin doses has been discussed in the previous chapter, but to do this successfully the pump user needs to understand what individual blood glucose results mean. When using a pump, the test results are a measure of how successfully the insulin delivered over the past few hours has affected the blood glucose. One of the most important aspects is to compare blood glucose readings over time, rather than to assess individual readings. Examples of how this can be used in practice are shown in Table 11.2, which shows how frequent testing, leaving only a few hours between each test, can help someone new to pump use understand their blood glucose readings and therefore make precise and often small adjustments to their insulin doses.

# Glycaemic targets to aim for

For the first few days of using an insulin pump, achieving good glycaemic control is not the aim. Avoiding hypoglycaemia is the first priority, and the second is to try and obtain some stability and to avoid, or reduce the number of, major fluctuations in blood glucose levels. The pump user will still have some long-acting insulin influencing their blood glucose levels in the first day or two, and also they are learning how to manage their diabetes in a different way, so gaining confidence with using the pump is a bigger priority than glycaemic control.

The pump user's pre-pump blood glucose levels, the difficulties they were having prior to using a pump and their personal views should all have some bearing on the initial glycaemic targets set. Examples of how targets might be set can be seen in Table 11.3. In all the examples shown, the target ranges are unlikely to be those aimed for in the long term, but they will help the pump user avoid hypoglycaemia and also give them a target to aim for with correction

**Table 11.3**  Setting initial glycaemic targets

| Prior to using a pump | Initial glycaemic targets |
|---|---|
| hypoglycaemia most days, loss of warning signs and symptoms, wants to keep blood glucose high | 8–15 mmol/l: avoid hypoglycaemia at all times |
| retinopathy developing as a result of poor glycaemic control | avoid tight control initially as it could worsen retinopathy: possibly aim for 8–14 mmol/l |
| swinging blood glucose readings between 3 and 20 mmol/l | aim for stability only, possibly within a wide range, 6–14 mmol/l |
| blood glucose levels usually below 10 but occasional hypos and readings over 20 mmol/l | aim for stability and avoid hypoglycaemia, 6–10 mmol/l |

boluses. It is important not to instil a sense of failure at this point: many people have high hopes when starting a pump and expect good glycaemic control very quickly, and so find it is hard to understand why they should not aim for this immediately. Others are fearful of hypoglycaemia and can be wary of reducing their blood glucose level below 10 mmol/l (millimoles per litre) in case it suddenly drops a lot lower. Having a slightly higher range to aim for means that if they over- or underestimate the effect of something, such as food or activity, they will not immediately experience hypoglycaemia. Also, some people experience major variations in their blood glucose level in the first few days, as their body adjusts to insulin being delivered in a very precise way, but once this period is over it will become possible to start to closely adjust the insulin doses.

Once some stability has been gained by adjusting insulin doses, the target blood glucose level can be gradually reduced, possibly by a millimole or two every few days. Some people might gain good glycaemic control within the first week, particularly if their glycaemic control was reasonable before they started using a pump. For the majority, it is likely to be three or four weeks before they reach their final target range, and for those whose adjustment is slower it might be a number of months before this is achieved.

The long-term aim should be close to normoglycaemia, with blood glucose levels of 4–7 mmol/l and an HbA1c level below seven per cent without frequent hypoglycaemia, although these targets might vary for some individuals, depending on their circumstances. If someone is pregnant, tighter glycaemic control will be aimed for. Likewise, if complications are already present, the aim might be to achieve much tighter control, based on the evidence from the Diabetes Control and Complications Trial Research Group (1993) that tight control can minimise the risk of the progression of existing complications.

# Record-keeping

Reviewing the success of insulin pump therapy is made much easier if detailed records are kept. The aim of record-keeping is to develop a system that will help the pump user in the long term, rather than simply one that is used as a reporting system. Health professionals might initially be involved in troubleshooting and analysing the records brought to the clinic, but this should always be done with the pump user, who should be encouraged to give their opinions on the causes of any blood glucose fluctuations, how successful their management has been and what action they might consider taking in the future. The more pump users are involved, the more opportunity there will be to assess their understanding and decision-making ability.

Standard information that is helpful to collect includes:

- dates and times for all of the information recorded
- blood glucose levels
- type of food eaten and its carbohydrate content
- all insulin boluses, including correction boluses, the total amounts and what type of bolus was used
- any episodes of hypoglycaemia or hyperglycaemia and how it was treated
- any symptoms of hypoglycaemia or hyperglycaemia (and the blood glucose levels at the time)
- any temporary basal rates and how long they were used for
- any changes made to basal rates or to bolus ratios
- any specific situations (e.g. physical activity) and actions taken to deal with them
- the effect of alcohol on blood glucose values and the management strategies used
- any time when the pump has been removed
- when the infusion set and site have been changed.

The information gathered as above helps the pump user to understand the impact of different actions on their blood glucose levels, to make dose and lifestyle adjustments and to plan what strategies will be most successful when dealing with similar situations in the future.

On a longer-term basis, most pump users will decide for themselves what written records they want to keep. They are likely to very quickly stop writing down the food they eat and might stop recording their blood glucose readings because their meter has a memory, and they might not record changes they've made to their basal rate. While this is because they are growing in confidence and don't need to write everything down to know whether it is working for them, when attending a clinic appointment it can be more difficult to identify what proactive management decisions would help. It might be possible to develop a system or agreement with pump users about what needs to be regularly written down and also what information it would be useful to bring to a clinic appointment to make the best use of the time. If there are specific aims and targets that the pump user is trying to achieve, the record-keeping could be geared towards collecting that information.

## Using records in a consultation

Consultations should be viewed as a joint sharing of expertise. Health professionals who specialise in insulin pump therapy will be able to bring their factual knowledge and experience to the consultation, but the pump user is also a rich source of information, particularly when assessing the success of self-management. A questioning approach is helpful, to elicit what thought processes informed the decisions that were made. Questions that might be useful in a consultation include:

- What have your blood glucose levels been like?
- Where have they been within your target range and when have they been outside it?
- When they are outside the range, what causes that?
- What action did you take at the time?
- Do you think anything needs altering – or have you altered anything – to prevent it happening again?
- Can you explain to me how you managed xxxx situation?

It could be helpful to share the above questions with the pump user so that they know what will be useful information to bring to the consultation, and also so that they can develop their own process along similar lines to deal with any blood glucose levels they are not happy with.

## Using computer data systems

Many pumps now have computer software that is either accessible via the Internet or can be bought and loaded on to a computer (as discussed in more detail in Chapter Four). Much of the information discussed in this chapter can be stored on computer and emailed to health professionals, kept on home computer systems or downloaded in a clinic setting. This can be useful for some people, especially if they enjoy using computers and if the information helps them see trends and make choices they might otherwise not have done. However, it is also important to recognise that not all pump users will want such detailed analysis and might not find the time to do it or might feel that this makes their diabetes more intrusive than it would otherwise have been.

If computer data are used as part of the review process, it is important to keep the principles of successful consultations in mind, as already outlined, namely that the pump user, rather than the health professional, should be the person who is identifying where things are working well and what action can be taken to address the areas which are not as successful. It is also important not to simply look at average results, as this does not allow for the identification of variations in daily routines and specific situations that have caused a high or low blood glucose reading.

## HYPOGLYCAEMIA

The avoidance of hypoglycaemia, or a reduction in its frequency, is a common reason for someone wishing to start using an insulin pump. Studies have demonstrated that not only is this achievable but that, when people do experience hypoglycaemia, it happens much more gradually and also that the symptoms of hypoglycaemia can be felt at a much higher blood glucose level than pre-pump (Everett, 2003). Anecdotally, people also report that they feel more in control, as they are aware of when things start to go wrong and can therefore deal with it much more quickly, which reduces anxiety.

### Symptoms of hypoglycaemia

When someone starts to use a pump, they can find that their hypoglycaemia symptoms are different from those previously experienced or that they have regained more awareness of when hypoglycaemia is occurring. This might be due to the reduction in extreme blood glucose swings that most people can achieve or because of changes in their counter-regulatory hormone responses. The lack of subcutaneous depots of longer-acting insulin is also likely to play a part. As the hypoglycaemic episodes are less frequent, many of the early symptoms of hypoglycaemia can return, such as shakiness and sweating, and pump users usually experience these symptoms when their blood glucose level is still above 3 mmol/l. Treating their hypoglycaemic episode at this stage avoids the later symptoms developing.

### Causes of hypoglycaemia

The simple reason why people experience hypoglycaemia is because they have more insulin acting than they need. There are a multitude of reasons for this,

**Table 11.4**  Causes of hypoglycaemia when using insulin pumps

| Causes | Examples |
|---|---|
| Too much insulin in the form of boluses | • the amount of insulin given for a food bolus was too large, either from overestimating the carbohydrate content of a meal or snack, giving a large bolus rather than an extended or split bolus, or from a mathematical error<br>• a bolus has been given twice in error<br>• too many correction doses have been given in a short space of time or too high a correction dose has been calculated |
| The insulin dose hasn't been reduced as it should have been | • insulin doses have not been decreased or extra carbohydrate has not been eaten when alcohol has been consumed<br>• the basal rate is set too high or hasn't been adjusted to take account of lower insulin requirements<br>• increased physical activity has been undertaken without either insulin doses being decreased or extra carbohydrate being eaten<br>• insulin hasn't been reduced enough to take into account the delayed effect of physical activity on reducing blood glucose levels<br>• the pump user has not reduced their insulin dose to account for other causes of hypoglycaemia, such as hot weather or stress in some people |
| Programming is inappropriate for the situation | • a temporary increased basal rate has been set too high or has been set but is no longer required, and has not been switched off |
| Other reasons | • there has been a longer timescale than anticipated between giving a bolus and eating<br>• the clock on the pump is wrong, giving the wrong basal rate for the time of day<br>• the infusion set has been primed while the pump is still connected to the cannula in the body |

some related to general diabetes management and others directly relating to pump use, which are listed in Table 11.4.

## Treatment of hypoglycaemia

As with any episode of hypoglycaemia, immediate treatment should be encouraged, by taking 10 grams of fast-acting carbohydrate, such as a glucose drink, glucose tablets or glucose gel, and without an insulin bolus being given.

The blood glucose should also be tested, as symptoms can change and might not be a reliable indicator of the blood glucose level. Following the intake of carbohydrate, the blood glucose should be checked 10 minutes later, and, if it is still below 4 mmol/l, a second 10 grams of fast-acting carbohydrate should be taken. Unlike with injection therapy, in most cases longer-acting carbohydrate is not required, as there is no long-acting insulin and therefore there is much less risk of hypoglycaemia recurring once it has been treated.

Opinions vary regarding whether the insulin dose should be stopped for a short period or whether the basal rate should be reduced. Some pump users might wish to stop their insulin if they experience hypoglycaemia; if this is the case, they should be advised to switch the pump off for no longer than 30 minutes, as the cumulative effect of less insulin plus extra carbohydrates can result in a raised blood glucose level an hour or two later. An alternative to switching off the pump is to programme a temporary basal rate reduction so that a small amount of insulin is still being delivered. However, many pump users find that additional carbohydrate alone will be enough to treat the hypoglycaemic episode, without altering their insulin dose.

If severe hypoglycaemia is experienced, so the pump user is unable to act or is unconscious, the insulin should be stopped temporarily. This should be done by either switching the pump off or disconnecting the infusion set, *not* by removing the cannula or cutting the tubing, as this would mean that the insulin could not be reconnected easily. An injection of glucagon should be administered, as it would be for people with diabetes using injection therapy. The hypoglycaemic effects would be expected to wear off quickly following the injection and the interruption to the insulin infusion. Once the blood glucose has risen to within the target range, insulin can start to be infused again.

In relation to severe hypoglycaemia, friends, relatives and colleagues should be aware of what action to take, as they might be inclined to remove the cannula or cut the tubing. The pump user should be able to identify the key people that need to learn how to stop the pump in an emergency, and might also consider providing written instructions, for example when at work, to ensure severe hypoglycaemia is dealt with correctly. In reality, severe hypoglycaemia is much rarer when using pump therapy, but someone who has experienced this in the past is likely to be anxious about it, and a clear plan of what to do will help reduce their anxiety.

Once the pump user has recovered from the hypoglycaemic episode, if they are about to eat a meal they should consider reducing their food bolus by 0.5 to 1 units to avoid further hypoglycaemia. Also, as with injection therapy, they should wait at least 30 minutes, and recheck their blood glucose level, before driving.

## Prevention of hypoglycaemia

As well as treating hypoglycaemic episodes, being aware of their causes and taking steps to address these will reduce the risk of their recurrence. The following steps can help pump users to avoid hypoglycaemia developing:

- Reduce insulin doses in situations that might cause low blood glucose readings (e.g. during and after physical activity or when consuming alcohol).
- Use different ways of giving boluses with high-carbohydrate or high-fat meals, rather than giving all the insulin as a standard bolus.
- Regularly assess the insulin to carbohydrate ratio and how successful it is, and adjust if necessary.
- Ensure the basal rate is assessed regularly, and adjust if necessary.
- Try and avoid miscalculations in bolus amounts for both food and correcting high blood glucose levels.
- Be aware of their symptoms and treat promptly.
- Take blood glucose readings before situations when hypoglycaemia can cause additional problems (e.g. when driving or before bed).
- Regularly review blood glucose results, including taking readings during the night at least once a month, to ensure glycaemic targets are being met.
- Review the results of any changes made to insulin doses.

## HYPERGLYCAEMIA

Insulin pumps deliver rapid-acting or short-acting insulin only, with no longer-acting insulin being given. This means that, if the insulin supply is insufficient or is interrupted, hyperglycaemia is likely to have a more rapid onset than when using injection therapy. Research has identified that knowledgeable and motivated pump users do not develop ketoacidosis more frequently than when using injection therapy, but prompt action is still required to avoid the risk of this developing.

Once good glycaemic control is established, as with hypoglycaemia, pump users are likely to experience symptoms relating to high blood glucose levels at an earlier stage. Whereas prior to using a pump they might have regularly had blood glucose levels of 15 mmol/l or above, they can feel quite unwell if their blood glucose now rises to around 10 or 11 mmol/l. This is probably due to their becoming accustomed to blood glucose levels fluctuating less than when injection therapy was used.

# Causes of hyperglycaemia

Hyperglycaemia will occur when insufficient insulin has been delivered to keep the blood glucose level well controlled. This can be for a number of reasons, which are listed in Table 11.5. It is important that pump users are aware of the different situations when hyperglycaemia can occur, as many of them are specific to pump use. This will equip them to identify and promptly rectify any causes of hypoglycaemia if it occurs, before it becomes a more major problem.

**Table 11.5**   Causes of hyperglycaemia when using insulin pumps

| | |
|---|---|
| Too little insulin has been given in the form of boluses | • the amount of insulin given for a food bolus was too small, either from underestimating the carbohydrate content of a meal or snack or from a mathematical error<br>• less insulin has been delivered by mistake, such as forgetting to give a meal/snack bolus or splitting the bolus and forgetting to give the second half |
| Basal rates have not been increased when required | • the basal rate is set too low<br>• insulin requirements have increased (e.g. around the time of menstruation, during pregnancy, when unwell, when infection is present, when steroids are taken or less physical activity than usual is being undertaken) |
| Difficulties with the infusion site | • insulin is not being delivered, from the cannula being dislodged or kinked, blood blocking the cannula or the infusion set leaking<br>• insulin is not being absorbed properly, from the cannula being inserted incorrectly or inserted into an area where absorption is reduced, such as scar tissue or areas of lipohypertrophy<br>• the site of the cannula is inflamed or infected from not changing the site frequently enough, not paying enough attention to hygiene when changing the infusion set or from oversensitivity to the plaster, the needle or the insulin |
| Other causes | • air is being infused, either from a large air bubble in the infusion set or from not priming the infusion set fully<br>• the insulin is out of date or has been exposed to high temperatures or has been frozen<br>• the pump has been in stop mode or disconnected for too long<br>• the pump is malfunctioning |

# Treatment of hyperglycaemia

The initial treatment of any hyperglycaemia is to give a correction bolus. This should be given whenever the blood glucose level is higher than the target range, even if it is only 1 or 2 mmol/l higher, and the blood glucose should be retested two hours later. The pump and the cannula insertion site should also be checked to ensure that insulin is being delivered. If the blood glucose level is still elevated two hours later, but has improved, a second correction dose should be given via the pump. If, however, the glucose level has risen further, the second correction dose should be given using a syringe or insulin pen rather than the pump, and a new cannula inserted and attached to the pump. This is because the additional rise in blood glucose levels suggests that insulin is possibly not being delivered or not being absorbed from the site of the cannula.

If the blood glucose level is 5 mmol/l or more higher than the target range at any point, ketones should also be checked for, ideally using a meter that checks blood ketone levels or by urine testing. If more than a trace of ketones is present, the amount of insulin given as a correction bolus should be doubled, as the usual correction dose is unlikely to be effective enough. In addition, the pump user should drink at least 500 millilitres of water per hour, to keep hydrated, and avoid excessive physical activity.

If hyperglycaemia persists, the pump user should contact their diabetes team for further advice. If nausea and vomiting occur, they should seek emergency medical help, either from their GP or from the local accident and emergency department, as ketoacidosis can quickly develop. More information about the management of illness and ketoacidosis can be found in Chapter 15.

Blood glucose tests can be carried out more frequently than two-hourly, particularly if the pump user is feeling unwell and is concerned about how high their blood glucose is, but correction boluses should be given no closer than one and a half hours apart, and ideally two hours apart. This is to avoid overcorrection by giving additional insulin before the initial correction bolus has taken full effect; otherwise, hypoglycaemia can occur.

As well as treating hyperglycaemia, it is also important for the pump user to analyse the cause of the hyperglycaemia. If illness is the cause, for example, it is likely that ongoing correction boluses will be needed, and a temporary increase in the basal rate will also help. If the hyperglycaemia is caused by a forgotten meal bolus, it is likely to be easily resolved with one or two correction boluses. If it is not possible to establish a cause, the pump user should make careful checks of the pump, tubing and cannula and, if in doubt, should change the infusion site and/or the infusion set to ensure that insulin is being delivered.

## Prevention of hyperglycaemia

Regular blood glucose testing will help to ensure that high blood glucose readings are identified early so that prompt action can be taken. The initial education package should raise the pump user's awareness of the importance of this, as well as the recognition that the presence of ketones indicates that more urgent action is required, and this should be reinforced at future appointments.

Other steps that can be taken to prevent hyperglycaemia developing, or to treat it early enough, are:

- ensuring the basal rate and the insulin to carbohydrate ratios are effective in controlling the blood glucose level
- changing the infusion set and the cannula at the recommended intervals, using good hygiene when doing so
- inspecting the infusion site at least daily
- regularly checking the tubing for any air bubbles
- increasing basal rates and insulin doses when unwell or inactive
- giving correction doses as soon as hyperglycaemia is detected, and monitoring the effects of these
- carrying emergency supplies (see Chapter 12).

## CONCLUSION

This chapter has outlined the general considerations involved in gaining optimum glycaemic control when using a pump. These include monitoring blood glucose levels, keeping records and dealing with the risk of hypoglycaemia and hyperglycaemia. This information, together with knowledge about making specific adjustments to insulin doses discussed in the previous chapter, will help pump users develop skills and strategies to manage their pump therapy in the longer term.

## REFERENCES

Diabetes Control and Complications Trial Research Group (1993) The effect of intensive treatment of diabetes on the development and progression of long-term complications in insulin-dependent diabetes mellitus. *New England Journal of Medicine* **329**(14): 977–986.

Everett J (2003) Insulin pump therapy: Where are we now? *Journal of Diabetes Nursing* **7**(6): 232–235.

Chapter 12
# The Day-to-day Management of Insulin Pump Therapy

This chapter provides information on dealing with various situations in which specific action might be needed in relation to insulin pump therapy. First, management of infusion sets and care of the infusion site are discussed, followed by how the pump can be worn and then information on what supplies to have available at all times is given. How to safely remove the pump for short or longer periods and dealing with physical activity, including sexual activity, are then outlined. Finally, how to plan for successful holidays and travel when using a pump is covered.

The information in this chapter should be used as general guidance, as different people prefer to manage situations in different ways. It is important to find solutions that work for pump users rather than providing blanket information and rules. For example, there are many different ways of giving additional insulin when required, and also of reducing insulin doses. Involving the pump user in choosing what action to take, experimenting to see whether their plan of action works for them and discussing what changes to make are the methods most likely to help them develop long-term coping and decision-making strategies.

## MANAGING INFUSION SETS AND SITES

Ensuring that the infusion site is looked after properly will greatly reduce the chances of infection and alteration in insulin absorption, both of which are likely to make it more difficult to achieve good glycaemic control.

### Siting of the infusion set

Options of where a needle or cannula can be sited are outlined in Table 12.1. The abdomen is the preferred site to use, as insulin absorption is fastest and

**Table 12.1**  Recommended infusion sites

1. **Abdominal area:** at least 2 cm from the umbilicus and 2 cm away from any scars or stretch marks. Can be sited both above and below the umbilicus and across the whole abdominal area.
2. **Buttocks:** upper outer quadrant
3. **Thighs:** mid- to upper outer thighs

most predictable and is unlikely to be affected by physical activity. The thigh or buttock areas are preferred by some, and practically might be the best option for them, but if activity is undertaken involving the muscles in those areas the insulin can be absorbed more rapidly and cause fluctuations in blood glucose levels. The abdomen is also more easily accessible and allows the infusion site to be checked visually by the pump user. The exact siting depends on personal preference but also on what clothing is worn, for example avoiding areas such as under a waistband.

Siting the infusion set is a skill that develops with practice, and the manufacturer's instructions should be closely followed. Pinching up the skin in the chosen area can help, but this will not always be possible as it will depend on which site the pump user has chosen. The infusion sets with Teflon cannulae can be slightly more difficult to insert because of the thickness of the cannula, but this will become easier with practice. Some pumps have an automatic insertion device that might help (see Chapter Four for more information). Also, some pump and infusion set manufacturers recommend that a 0.5 unit bolus of insulin is given when a cannula is first inserted, to fill the space created when the needle is removed.

## Changing the infusion set

For most pump users, the infusion site needs to be changed every two to three days, depending on the cannula type, to maintain consistent insulin absorption and also to minimise the chances of an infection developing. If absorption is poor or the site is beginning to become infected, blood glucose levels are likely to rise, which would indicate that the site needs changing. Some pump users find more frequent site changes, such as every 24 hours, are needed to maintain good glycaemic control.

When changing the infusion set or cannula, good hygiene principles should be followed. The area chosen should be dry and clean and hands should be washed prior to handling the infusion set. Changing the infusion site after a bath or shower in the morning is ideal. Inserting a new cannula late in the evening should be avoided, as it is important to check the blood glucose level two hours later to ensure that insulin is being absorbed from the new site.

If pump users begin to experience redness at the infusion site, or it becomes infected on more than one occasion, they should take greater hygiene precautions, which could simply be more thorough washing and drying, but some might also need to use antiseptic handwash and antiseptic wipes to clean the skin before inserting a new cannula. If an infection does occur, the infusion site should be changed immediately and the infection treated with antibiotics.

If desired, when first learning how to change the cannula, the old one can be kept in place until the new one is inserted. This is because the initial cannula changes that pump users carry out at home can be a time of high anxiety, and, if they find it difficult to insert the new cannula, pump users can experience feelings of panic. If the old cannula is still in place, insulin can still be infused and the pump user has plenty of time to insert the new one, then, once they are happy that the new one is in place, insulin can start to be infused through it. Anecdotally, pump users have found great reassurance in using this method, and some prefer to keep the old cannula in place for a further two hours to give them time to check their blood glucose level to ensure that insulin is being infused properly at the new site.

Some people find they experience lipohypertrophy when using a pump. If infusion areas become hard, or swollen, or lipohypertrophy is suspected, the site should be avoided until this has subsided, which is likely to take many months or, in some cases, years. Other difficulties can be allergies to the tape attached to the cannula. If this is suspected, the pump user can try a different dressing next to their skin, for example a film or hydrocolloid dressing, and can then insert the cannula through the dressing.

## WEARING THE PUMP

A new pump is likely to have one or two pouches or clips for attaching the pump to clothing, and others can be obtained either from the manufacturer or from other sources (see the Appendix for more information). Many potential pump users have concerns about where they will wear the pump and what to do with it in different situations. Ensuring it is accessible when required, but also that it doesn't get in the way and that the tubing won't get caught on door handles or furniture, is a challenge. This section looks at the different options of where and how the pump can be worn.

### Clipped or attached to a waistband

This is the most common place for insulin pumps to be worn, as the pump is easily accessible when it is required, and is also usually close to the infusion site so the tubing can often easily be tucked under clothes and is unlikely to catch on door handles or furniture. The pump user can wear it in front of their body, to the side or at the back. Some cases have clips that can be used to attach the pump to clothing or a loop to allow a strap or belt to be threaded through the back of the case. If the pump is attached securely to the waistband of trousers, it needs to be remembered and managed carefully when going to the toilet or when the trousers are taken off.

## Tucked into clothes

Insulin pumps can be put in trouser pockets and shirt pockets, which makes them easily retrievable and also avoids the need for a separate case for the pump. Some pump users make small holes in the back of their pockets so that the tubing can be threaded through and attached to the pump, rather than the tubing being external. This makes it more discreet and also reduces the potential of catching the tubing. Pumps can also be tucked into underwear (down the centre of a bra or into pants), although care needs to be taken with hygiene, and also it is important to be able to retrieve the pump for when boluses need to be given.

## On the arm or leg

Small straps can be used to attach the pump to the upper arm, which might be useful if sports are being played. A thigh strap is also an option, which can help if a dress is being worn that has no obvious place to attach the pump, or it can be worn under trousers. It can also be clipped on to the top of a boot, under trousers, as long as the tubing is long enough to reach to the infusion site, and can then be hidden and used discreetly.

## Sewing pouches into clothes

This might be the preferred option, although it takes time and commitment from the pump user to create their pouches. It can be useful for clothes that have no obvious place to put the pump, and can also be useful for nightwear.

## During the night

The pump does not have to be secured in bed, but, if the pump user prefers that it is, pockets or pouches in pyjamas and nightdresses are useful or the pump can be strapped to an arm, a leg or a strap round the waist. Many pump users do not secure their pump during the night; instead, they either tuck it under the pillow or simply leave it loose in the bed. This can raise concerns that it might be dislodged during the night, but anecdotally it tends to remain secure, although needs to be remembered if getting out of bed during the night for any reason.

## Securing the pump for sports

Pumps need to be more secure when undertaking certain sports or strenuous activities. Clip cases are not recommended, as they might easily become dislodged. Pouches that allow a strap to be threaded through the case are more secure, and also wearing them under clothes can prevent them being accidentally dislodged. The pump should be removed if contact sports, such as judo or rugby, are undertaken, as discussed later in this chapter.

## Summary

There are many different places that a pump can be worn. Choices will depend on how accessible the pump needs to be in different situations, and also on how comfortable the pump user is with having their pump on display. While many people now carry mobile phones, and pagers are common, an insulin pump can still carry some stigma and make pump users feel self-conscious. Discussing the options before pump therapy is initiated will be useful for some, and helping them find ways to wear the pump without embarrassment or inconvenience is an important part of integrating pump therapy into their lives.

## DAY-TO-DAY SUPPLIES

Because an insulin pump delivers rapid- or short-acting insulin only, if this is insufficient or interrupted, action needs to be taken quickly to avoid hyperglycaemia, which could potentially lead to ketoacidosis. It is therefore essential to ensure that there are adequate supplies available at all times in case things go wrong. As a minimum, it is recommended that pump users carry with them:

- blood glucose testing equipment, to be able to check blood glucose levels whenever necessary
- spare batteries for the pump, as the batteries might expire within a few hours of the 'low battery' alarm sounding on a pump

- an insulin syringe, or an insulin pen, needles and a spare insulin cartridge, to be able to give insulin by alternative means in an emergency
- a spare infusion set and tape, so that the infusion set and site can be changed if blood glucose levels start to rise
- ketone testing equipment, in case of hyperglycaemia
- glucose or equivalent, in case of hypoglycaemia.

Regarding whether to carry an insulin syringe or insulin pen, many pump users find a syringe much easier to carry around than an insulin pen, because of its size, and it might be possible to fit the syringe, plus the other equipment listed above, into the wallet of a blood glucose meter. With a syringe, insulin can be drawn straight from the cartridge in the pump if required. It is useful to check that the pump user is familiar with using syringes, as many people use an insulin pen from diagnosis. If an insulin pen is carried, it is also important to carry an insulin cartridge and needles to fit the pen.

In some circumstances, a spare supply of insulin for the pump might also need to be carried. The pumps have alarm systems that alert the pump user to their insulin supply getting low, usually when around 20 units are left, although this is variable depending on the type of pump used. Many people use less than 20 units per day, and therefore might feel confident that they will not need additional supplies, but they could use more than anticipated if, for example, they needed to prime a new infusion set. Helping them to plan ahead regarding how they will manage this situation will help to avoid the pump user being without insulin. They could, for example, keep a spare supply in the refrigerator at work or at someone's house if they regularly visit, or at school if they are a pupil. If spare supplies are kept, their expiry dates should be checked regularly, and they should be replenished as soon as possible if they are used. It is also useful to remind pump users that insulin should only be left out of the refrigerator for one month, so spare supplies should be kept in a refrigerator whenever possible.

If for any reason it is not possible to use the pump to deliver insulin, insulin will need to be injected using either a syringe or pen. It is possible to inject the rapid-acting insulin analogue from the pump in an emergency, which would need to be injected at two- to three-hourly intervals to ensure enough insulin is in the pump user's body. For longer periods, conversion to multiple-dose insulin therapy will be necessary, as discussed later in this chapter. Because this might be needed, pump users should be encouraged to keep a supply of longer-acting insulin, such as isophane or a long-acting insulin analogue, and also a spare insulin pen or syringe. This insulin should be kept in their refrigerator, and the expiry date should be checked regularly.

## REMOVING THE PUMP FOR SHORT PERIODS

It is possible to take the pump off temporarily, for a maximum of two hours at any one time, but shorter periods are recommended as they are easier to manage. The action to take will depend on why the pump has been taken off, and what is expected to happen to the blood glucose levels during that time. Examples are:

- when showering or bathing
- when swimming
- when undertaking rough or contact sports
- when undertaking sexual activity
- when using a sauna or jacuzzi
- when undergoing minor hospital procedures, such as X-rays or scans.

Short breaks of around 20 to 30 minutes are unlikely to make a great deal of difference to the pump user's blood glucose levels. If the pump is taken off for an hour, the pump user should check their blood glucose levels when they recommence using the pump, and give a correction bolus if necessary. If the blood glucose levels are within the target range and no correction bolus is required, they should be checked again an hour later, as the lack of insulin can have a longer effect and a correction bolus might be needed at this point.

If the pump has been off for the maximum time of two hours, it is highly likely that some degree of hyperglycaemia will occur, and a correction dose should be given when the pump is reconnected. This dose can be determined by the blood glucose level at the time, but this might be insufficient as the blood glucose is likely to be rising, so a second correction dose might be needed two hours later. If the pump has been taken off for physical activity, correction boluses are less likely to be needed, particularly if the activity has been intense or has lasted a long time (see the 'Physical activity' section later in this chapter for more information).

The basal rate at the time the pump is removed should also be taken into consideration. If a high basal rate is being infused at the time, a larger proportion of the pump user's total daily insulin dose will be missed, increasing the likelihood of a correction bolus being needed when the pump is reconnected. Over time, the pump user will learn what is likely to happen to their blood glucose level if they regularly have situations where the pump needs to be removed. They might then be able to prevent recurring hyperglycaemia by identifying what bolus dose of insulin they need when they reconnect to the pump.

In reality, pump users will use a variety of techniques to manage their insulin doses when removing the pump, particularly if the reason for removal is a regular occurrence for them. Giving a small bolus before removing the pump is an option some people will choose to avoid hyperglycaemia. If a longer period of disconnection is required, this could be managed by the pump being reconnected at intervals of no more than two hours, a bolus being given and the pump then being disconnected again.

## REMOVING THE PUMP FOR LONG PERIODS

Part of the initial education package should include how someone should manage if they need to disconnect the pump for a long period of time, either through choice or if circumstances determine that this is necessary. Choosing to stop using the pump might include times when someone feels they want a break from wearing it every day or if they feel they no longer want to continue with pump therapy. Circumstances where it might be necessary to remove the pump might be if it malfunctions and it is not possible to get a replacement pump for a few days.

Whatever the reason, the pump user needs to be able to calculate how much insulin they need to give if they revert to using multiple-dose insulin therapy. They are likely to need a larger amount of insulin using injection therapy, so they should total up their average total daily insulin dose on the pump and add 20 per cent to it, which will give them a new total to use as a basis for their injection therapy. This can then be split as the pump user wishes (the most straightforward way is to divide it into four equal doses, one for the longer-acting insulin and three meal bolus doses). They will probably continue assessing their carbohydrate intake and giving insulin to match and so are unlikely to use the fixed mealtime doses, but they might be useful as a starting point.

As with any change in the insulin regimen, pump users will need to use their blood glucose monitoring results to assess their basal insulin and their mealtime insulin to carbohydrate ratio, and are likely to need to make adjustments. If the pump is only being removed for a few days, this might not be too important, but it will be required for longer periods.

## PHYSICAL ACTIVITY

As with other aspects of insulin pump therapy, managing physical activity is approached by trying to mimic the body's natural insulin requirements. Activity causes glycogen to be released from the liver, which is converted into glucose to meet the additional energy requirements of the muscles. As activity continues, this glucose is used by the muscles and blood glucose levels will start to fall. If the activity is fairly intense or of a long duration, the blood glucose might also fall during the few hours following the activity, and for strenuous exercise, blood glucose levels can take 24 hours to return to normal, owing to glucose being taken from the blood to replace the glycogen used from the liver.

Trying to develop a management plan that will closely match the insulin requirements for different types of activity is a challenge, and an experimental approach should be used to try and identify the best way of managing blood glucose levels. When using injection therapy, it is difficult or sometimes impossible to reduce the insulin in an effective way, so there is no choice but to increase the amount of carbohydrate eaten. For pump users, it is much easier to reduce the insulin dose precisely when it is required, although it is still possible, and sometimes necessary, to eat more carbohydrates instead of, or as an addition to, reducing insulin doses.

Ways of reducing the insulin dose include reducing the basal rate, either before, during or after the activity, or a combination of these times. Another option is to remove the pump for a short period to interrupt the delivery of insulin, which might be necessary in any case for some types of activity. Also, any boluses given shortly before or after the activity can be reduced. If extra carbohydrates are going to be eaten, again this could be before, during or after the activity.

The first stage in any planning is to identify how fit the person is already, what type of activity is going to be undertaken and for how long. The fitter someone is, the more efficiently they will use their glucose stores, so less adjustment will be needed. Looking at the type of activity will help someone to identify how much energy they are likely to use, and the length of time they will be active can help them identify whether it will have a short- or longer-term effect on their blood glucose level. Table 12.2 gives examples of different types of activity.

## Light activity

Light activity is unlikely to have a significant effect on blood glucose levels, as the muscles will not use large amounts of glucose, although it can make some difference.

**Table 12.2** Examples of light, moderate and intense activity

| | |
|---|---|
| Light activity | 30 minutes' walking or leisurely cycling, 1 hour's supermarket shopping, housework or light gardening |
| Moderate activity | Playing golf, 30 minutes' running, 1 hour's swimming or tennis |
| Intense activity | 2 hours' football, tennis or swimming, 1 hour's vigorous cycling |

Setting the temporary basal rate at 70 per cent an hour prior to the activity and then returning to the usual basal rate at the end of the activity is likely to be sufficient to manage this. If the activity has not been planned and the basal rate cannot be reduced an hour before, eating 10 grams of carbohydrate and using a temporary basal rate of 70 per cent for the duration of the activity is recommended. As with planned activity, the basal rate can be returned to the usual rate at the end of the activity, and no changes need to be made to bolus doses.

## Moderate activity

With moderate activity, the muscles will need a greater supply of glucose, so changes are likely to be needed to both basal rates and insulin bolus doses. If the activity is planned, the basal rate should be reduced to 50 per cent an hour prior to the activity, and might need to be continued for an hour after the activity is finished. If the activity has a prolonged effect, a basal rate reduction to 80–90 per cent might also be needed for a further hour or two. For food boluses just before, during or within an hour following the activity, an altered insulin to carbohydrate ratio should be used. For example, if the usual ratio is one unit of insulin per 10 grams of carbohydrate, this could be altered to one unit per 15 grams.

## Intense activity

With intense activity, glucose will be used rapidly both during the activity and for a period of time afterwards, and will require careful management. The effect of intense activity is less easy to predict, and advice should be tailored to the individual's situation, including taking into account their previous experiences. If someone already regularly undertakes sporting or other strenuous activity before they start using an insulin pump, their existing strategies can be used as a starting point, although they should be analysed in relation to how effective they have been.

If the pump user has no previous experience of this type of activity, the basal rate should be reduced to 50 per cent in advance as for moderate activity, and food boluses are likely to need a greater reduction, possibly only giving half of their usual insulin boluses. If food is eaten during the activity, the person might only need a very small bolus or no bolus at all. A reduced basal rate should be continued after the activity, which should be set at around 70 to 80 per cent, and this could be required for up to 12 hours. For this type of activity during the evening, an overnight temporary basal rate reduction should always be used.

## Removal of insulin pump for activity

If the choice is made to remove the insulin pump, this should be done immediately prior to the activity, and it should not be left off for more than two hours without reconnection and additional boluses being given. Some pump users will choose to disconnect rather than reduce their basal rate, but in other cases it might be safer or more logical to remove the pump, such as when engaged in contact sports like judo and rugby. If the pump is removed for team sports, testing blood glucose levels at half-time and possibly having a smaller than usual bolus for a snack will help to reduce fluctuations in blood glucose levels.

If the pump has been removed, it should be reconnected once the activity has finished. A reduced basal rate following this might be required for moderate activity, and will definitely be required for intense activity, as already discussed. As with any physical activity, blood glucose monitoring will help individuals to identify whether their strategy has been successful or whether they need to make further changes in the future.

## Additional points

It is important to check blood glucose levels before activity, and also not to increase activity if blood glucose levels are above 11–12 mmol/l (millimoles per litre), as this indicates a shortage of insulin to deal with the glycogen that will be converted, so blood glucose levels are likely to further rise if activity is undertaken. A correction bolus of insulin should be given, and the blood glucose level should be rechecked to ensure it has dropped before activity is commenced. It is important not to undertake additional physical activity if the blood glucose is above 14 mmol/l or if ketones are present.

Additional carbohydrate might be required, and is especially likely to be required for activity over a period of more than an hour. Boluses should be given to match the carbohydrate, but reduced amounts might be needed, as already discussed. Snacks should be readily available in case hypoglycaemia occurs, both during the period of activity and for a number of hours later.

The information provided here in relation to physical activity is for general guidance only, and there is likely to be great variation between individuals. Blood glucose monitoring is paramount in establishing how a pump user reacts to differing activity levels. Testing before activity, during (if lasting longer than an hour) and frequent testing in the hours following anything more than light activity will provide information that can be used as a basis for discussion about what strategies are successful and what might need to be planned for the next time the activity is undertaken. Asking a pump user to document exactly how they managed their diabetes around the time of the activity ensures that assessments are based on accurate information, which can be used as a basis for future planning.

## SEXUAL ACTIVITY

Sexual activity should be considered a form of physical activity, as it is likely to have an effect on blood glucose levels. As sexual activity is often spontaneous, it is difficult to plan ahead, so using a temporary basal rate reduction in advance might not be practicable. Depending on personal preference, the pump can be either left on or taken off during sexual activity. Following the activity, eating 10 to 20 grams of carbohydrate without giving an insulin bolus is likely to be sufficient to avoid hypoglycaemia. If the pump has been removed, it is important to remember to reconnect it, and, if the time off the pump has been longer than 30 minutes, correction doses might be required, as discussed earlier in this chapter.

## HOLIDAYS AND TRAVEL

Planning in advance for holidays and travelling will mean that the pump user has enough supplies and knows what to do to make their trip easier. If staying in the United Kingdom, it is advisable to take more supplies than are expected to be needed on holiday, including extra blood glucose testing strips, long-acting insulin, insulin pens and needles, in case there is a need to revert to injection therapy, and ketone testing equipment.

If travelling abroad, the above measures should be adopted, but additional planning is also needed. First, supplies for the pump: if flying, all insulin and ideally the pump supplies should be carried in hand luggage, to avoid the potential for luggage being lost on the way. It is a good idea to contact the airline prior to the journey to check any restrictions they might have on what can be carried in hand luggage, as pump supplies can take up a large amount of room when travelling for a week or two. Pumps can safely be worn through airport scanning machines without setting the alarm off or damaging the pump, but it is a good idea for people to tell the airport staff that they are wearing a pump. It is also a good idea to take quite a few carbohydrate-rich snacks for the flight, in case there are any disruptions to the flight timetables or hypoglycaemia occurs. Additional information to take might be the name of the pump user's usual insulin plus the pump manufacturer's office in the country that is being visited. A medical certificate stating that the person is using an insulin pump, plus the supplies they need to carry, can be useful.

Once on board the plane, the pump user should inform the cabin crew that they are wearing an insulin pump, to avoid causing unnecessary alarm when they are pressing buttons or if the pump beeps or alarms.

Some people feel that they might like to have time off the pump when on holiday, as they feel that injection therapy will be easier to manage when away, although anecdotally they often later report that their holiday has been more difficult using injections instead of the pump. If they wish to try injections, it is recommended that they still take their pump and supplies with them so that they can revert to pump therapy when they are on holiday if they wish to.

If travelling across time zones, if the time difference is up to two hours, re-setting the clock on the pump to local time on arrival is likely to be sufficient to maintain blood glucose levels close to the target range. For bigger time differences, if the pump user is concerned about hypoglycaemia occurring because of the variations in their basal rate, a temporary basal rate reduction could be programmed into the pump. Whatever strategy is used, close monitoring of blood glucose levels will be required, and frequent insulin adjustments might be needed. For even short flights involving travel across time zones, blood glucose levels are likely to be variable for at least 24 hours following the flight, so it is prudent to aim for slightly higher blood glucose levels for a day or two.

## Holiday activities

While on holiday, hot and cold temperatures can have a major impact on glycaemic control. Hot weather is more likely to induce hypoglycaemia, and also there is a danger that the sun will heat up the infusion set tubing and alter the effect of the insulin. Care should be taken to position the cannula in a convenient place so that it will not be in direct sunlight, for example when on the beach, and also the tubing should be kept out of the sun, by putting either clothing or a beach towel over it. For cold holidays, such as skiing, the pump should be kept close to the body, underneath clothing, to try and maintain it at an even temperature.

If swimming, it is advisable to remove the pump, although some manufac-turers provide waterproof covers for their pumps. If the pump is removed, it is advisable not to leave it on the beach; although it would be of little use to others, it might seem an attractive piece of equipment and could be stolen. Disconnecting is possible if someone else is able to look after the pump, or it can be locked away, and it is also important to ensure that enough insulin is delivered, particularly if the pump user is frequently swimming (additional boluses might be needed to cover the time that the pump is removed). Also, extra care should be taken to make sure the tape is secure if it is frequently getting wet, and additional tape might be needed to prevent the cannula from being dislodged.

Finally, blood glucose levels should be checked frequently and remedial action taken if they are outside the individual's target range. Hot and cold weather, differing levels of activity, different foods being eaten and possibly a reduced stress level can all affect blood glucose levels, and pump users report that frequent monitoring is worthwhile as it helps them have confidence in their glycaemic control and therefore enjoy their travel more.

## CONCLUSION

This chapter has discussed a number of different situations that require careful management to maintain glycaemic control. Using the past experiences of the pump user and frequent blood glucose monitoring will identify the best way of managing situations that are likely to disrupt glycaemic control. Keeping records of actions taken and their success is useful for future reference, together with thoughts on how a situation could have been managed better. Each pump user is different, and finding what works best for them will be the best solution, as well as adding to their experiences and skills to apply to new situations in the future.

# Chapter 13
# Insulin Pumps in Babies, Children and Teenagers

This chapter will discuss the rationale for using insulin pump therapy in children and young people and identify specific considerations and areas where practice needs to vary from the way that insulin pump therapy is used in adults. It will provide practical information about how to approach dealing with specific situations, particularly those where parents are providing the majority of diabetes care but cannot always be present. Information in other sections of this book will still be applicable to children as well as adults, and the reader will be referred to it where necessary.

## THE EVIDENCE BASE AND QUALITY OF LIFE

As with adults, there is ample evidence to support the use of insulin pump therapy with babies, children and teenagers. HbA1c levels have been shown to improve, and also the frequency and severity of hypoglycaemia can be reduced (Boland et al., 1999; Bode et al., 1996; Hanas and Adolfsson, 2006). Pump therapy can also stabilise blood glucose levels by reducing the variability in blood glucose levels post-prandially (Heptulla et al., 2004) and can improve the glycaemic control of young people who experience recurrent diabetic ketoacidosis (Rodrigues et al., 2005). All of these benefits not only help children and young people in the short term but also contribute to reducing the potential for developing long-term complications in later years.

There are a number of physiological reasons why insulin pumps are particularly useful for children. One is that children generally exhibit a higher sensitivity to insulin, particularly young children, which can result in marked nocturnal hypoglycaemia when using conventional insulin delivery methods. Use in teenagers also has benefits, as following puberty many experience a marked rise in blood glucose levels in the early morning (often referred to as the 'dawn phenomenon'). Added to this, the hormonal changes that occur during adolescence, along with growth and development, make predicting insulin requirements more difficult, so a more flexible system of insulin delivery, that can be rapidly altered, promotes better glycaemic control.

Regarding quality of life for children and their parents, being able to eat a wide variety of foods and at varying times are advantages that help children be like their peers. This means they can avoid situations where they have to eat because of the action of their insulin; instead, they can simply give an insulin bolus before, during or after food. This is particularly useful with babies and toddlers, who might snack at varying times or refuse food when offered. It also means that physical activity, often carried out with very little pre-planning, can be catered for.

Many children – and their parents – report that the children feel much better once they are using an insulin pump instead of injection therapy. They are less likely to experience mood swings because of reduced fluctuations in their blood glucose level, and being able to eradicate night-time hypoglycaemia means they have less tendency to wake up feeling tired, unwell or irritable, as well as parents being less anxious about their child's safety. This often reflects in more harmony within families, children being better able to concentrate at school and, in teenagers, being able to cope more easily with diabetes (Boland *et al.*, 1999). In addition, children are able to do many things that would have caused difficulties when using injection therapy, such as sleeping over with friends, eating snacks at the cinema, having treats on special occasions, going to parties and eating the sort of food their friends are eating, without feeling guilty or experiencing large fluctuations in their blood glucose levels.

## PRE-PUMP EXPECTATIONS AND ASSESSMENT

If insulin pump therapy is being considered for a child, assessment criteria will to a great extent resemble those for adults (as outlined in Chapter Six). However, there are particular aspects of caring for children with diabetes that might suggest a pump would provide benefits for this age group. These include how well a child performs at school, whether their school attendance is affected by unstable diabetes or whether behavioural problems related to mealtimes arise. NICE guidance (2003) highlights that the early initiation of pump therapy in children can be beneficial, and in some specialist teams pumps are beginning to be used from diagnosis in babies and toddlers. This is in recognition of the complexity of management in children of very young ages, including the very small doses of insulin required, the need for flexibility and the number of boluses needed to match the frequent snacks recommended by the British Nutrition Foundation for all small children to ensure an adequate intake of high-energy foods (British Nutrition Foundation, 2004).

An important part of the assessment process is identifying what expectations both the parents and their child have of an insulin pump, and whether all of them appear motivated. It is also helpful to assess the family dynamics, as disharmony within a family can make it difficult for everyone to work cohesively together to help a child become confident with insulin pump therapy. In some cases, the parents could be keen for their child to have a pump as they see it as a way of 'sorting out' their diabetes, whereas their child might be less keen. Conversely, sometimes a child is the one who wants the pump but their parents have reservations.

Talking through the reality of pump therapy with everyone concerned, including siblings, and asking them specific questions about their expectations will ensure they have a realistic view of the benefits and also the drawbacks of using an insulin pump. Children could view a pump as something that will automatically control their blood glucose level and so will need to understand that regular blood glucose monitoring and adjustment of insulin doses will continue to be part of their daily lives. They might also perceive that they can eat whatever they like if they have a pump, but, while that might be true in principle, they will still need to heed parental guidance and be aware of the importance of eating healthily. Table 13.1 outlines the key questions that should be asked when assessing whether insulin pump therapy is the right treatment option for a child.

There is no lower age limit for use of an insulin pump, and babies of only a few weeks old can gain particular benefits from using a pump, as highlighted earlier. There are additional practicalities to consider with small babies, including the delivery of very small insulin doses and the siting of the infusion set, which will be discussed later in this chapter.

When preparing to start using a pump to treat a child with diabetes, it is useful for the parents, as well as the child, to wear a saline pump for a few days. This will help them gain confidence with the technology and also some insight into what it is like to wear a pump 24 hours a day. They can also find it useful to borrow a saline-filled pump when their child first starts using a pump containing insulin, so that the parents and also the child can safely practise carrying out different functions on the spare pump without the danger of accidentally giving additional insulin.

**Table 13.1**  Assessing whether insulin pump therapy will benefit a child

---

Do both the parents and child want the pump, or is one party keener than the other?

Are there clinical indications (as per NICE guidance) that suggest a pump will provide benefits?

Do the parents and child understand the benefits and drawbacks of insulin pump therapy?

Is there commitment to working hard to make insulin pump therapy a success?

---

# ROLES AND RESPONSIBILITIES

It is important to be clear about the roles and responsibilities of parents and children with regard to using an insulin pump. The following are general recommendations about how much responsibility a child should have in relation to their pump.

## Below three years old

If insulin pump therapy is being used for a baby or toddler below the age of three, the parents and any other carers should provide all the care their child needs and will be completely responsible for managing the pump. The child should not be expected to be involved at all. If a child of this age displays curiosity about the pump, their questions should be answered, but they should not be encouraged to press buttons or get involved in working the pump. Rather, it should be seen as something that is not to be tampered with, and features such as keylocks and basal rate locks should always be used to prevent accidental programming by the child.

## Three to five years old

This is the age when toddlers are likely to start to display more curiosity about their pump, in the same way that they are curious about the world around them. When a toddler begins to make choices about the clothes they wear and the food they eat, they are likely at this stage to show an interest in their pump and might want to be involved. While responsibility at this age still remains firmly with the parents, involving the child in a minor way can be useful (letting them handle the pump, press buttons with help or choose their infusion site or pump carrying case are all options). Involving children in this way can help them to feel they have some measure of control over their pump, which can help to reduce their anxiety. However, they should not be encouraged to have any responsibility for managing any aspect of pump therapy, including those listed above.

## Five to ten years old

Once a child is attending school full-time, one issue to be considered is how to manage the bolus doses they will need at lunchtime, as well as possibly for snacks during the day (see the section 'Insulin pumps at school' later in this chapter for more information). Children under seven years of age will still need supervision when giving bolus doses, from either their parents or school staff.

It is relatively common for young children to forget to give their insulin boluses, particularly when snacking, as with injection therapy they might not have given food boluses other than at mealtimes. Letting a child become involved with carrying out what functions they can, with supervision, and also checking the pump memory and set up afterwards will provide parents with reassurance and confidence in their child's handling of the pump. As with other aspects of daily life, such as cleaning teeth or brushing hair, parents will need to provide reminders to their child to give their insulin boluses.

Children of this age might also be interested in getting more involved with other aspects of their pump therapy, such as priming the infusion set and making alterations to their basal rate. It is possible to involve them in these aspects, but they should not be expected to carry out these tasks on their own without help and support, and any aspect they are involved in should always be supervised and checked for accuracy and safety.

Children are often able to grasp new technology more quickly than their parents and so might start to feel that they can be in charge of their pump. In reality, they will not be able to make the sophisticated decisions and calculations that are required around insulin doses or know how to deal with different situations and will still need a lot of input from their parents. They might start to learn how to carry out many of the pump functions, from priming a new infusion set to altering their basal rates, but this should all be under supervision, and the results of their programming should also be checked.

Asking a child of below 10 years of age to carry out any pump functions other than bolusing without supervision is giving them too much responsibility and can also result in blood glucose fluctuations because of inaccurate pump handling and management. It can be hard at this stage for parents to get the right balance between allowing the child some freedom and responsibility while making sure they are fully in the picture of what is happening.

## 11 to 13 years old

When a child is nearing secondary-school age, the responsibilities between them and their parents become less distinct. At this age, children should be giving their lunchtime insulin boluses at school, and also giving additional boluses if they have snacks at break times. They might also be gaining confidence and competence in changing and priming their infusion set and in the general programming of their pump.

The age at which a child is able to calculate the carbohydrate content of their food, and what bolus to give, can vary, but around 11 years old is a general guide, as this is the time when they will be taught decimal points, ratios and percentages at school. Practising on meals eaten with the family, and possibly situations where the family is eating away from home, can be a way for children to gain confidence in assessing their carbohydrate intake. Also, helping a child anticipate what sort of food they are likely to eat when their parents aren't present and identifying what tools they can use to assess or check the amount of carbohydrate they are eating are all steps towards increasing independence in this area. However, even if a child does become more independent, parents should still periodically check how this is working, and revisiting carbohydrate assessment at regular intervals can help.

## 14 to 16 years old

Teenage years are a time for experimentation, and many teenagers are likely to want to try out different ways of altering their insulin doses and programming their insulin pump to match different situations. Some teenagers might be keen to be more autonomous with their pump, particularly around decision-making regarding how much insulin to take. This can result in parents feeling excluded or expressing concerns and anxieties about what their child is doing with the pump and how they are managing their diabetes. The *National Service Framework for Diabetes* (Department of Health, 2001) highlights that family support and involvement throughout childhood and teenage years are important aspects of helping children cope with their diabetes.

To help the family provide the necessary support, an open relationship between the teenager and their parents should be encouraged, where they can discuss what is being tried, how well it is working and what might need to be changed, and open discussions held in a clinic setting can provide examples of how this can be put into practice. While the temptation is to encourage independence, a lack of parental involvement is likely to result in teenagers taking less care of their diabetes. It is generally advocated that families should be involved as long as possible, with a gradual transfer of responsibility, as this has been shown to improve metabolic control and self-care. Also, a teenager's peer group is important in providing emotional support, again improving self-care (Greene and Greene, 2005).

## The involvement of others

There might also be other people who need to gain confidence in using the pump, particularly for young children. These could include childminders, nursery staff and grandparents or other relatives who are regularly involved in caring for the child. It is also important to include siblings in helping with the pump: while they might not have a major role to play, involving siblings helps to prevent the child with diabetes becoming the focus of family attention and creates a better support network for the child using the pump.

Often, one parent will assume the main caring role and will learn the most about the pump, but every effort should be made to involve the wider family and any support networks. By sharing decisions about insulin doses and managing different situations, the potential for one parent to become over-anxious because of the responsibility they have is reduced. Involving, as far as possible, all significant people and family members when the initial pump training takes place will help them gain understanding and insight to help a child get the most from using their pump.

## SETTING INSULIN DOSE RATES

This section discusses how basal rates, food boluses and correction boluses should be initially set and also adjusted in younger age groups.

### Basal rates

When setting initial basal infusion rates, as with adults, the pre-pump insulin doses can be used as a starting point. The total amount of insulin given using injections should be totalled up and then reduced by around 30 per cent, to give the approximate amount of insulin that is likely to be required each day (referred to below as the 'total daily dose'). To determine how much of that total should be given as the basal rate depends on how old a child is – unlike adults, where 50 per cent is generally considered to be needed. The following can be used as guidelines regarding how much insulin should be given as the basal rate in children:

- Pre-school children: 35–40 per cent of the total daily dose
- Pubescent children: 40–45 per cent of the total daily dose
- Teenagers: up to 60 per cent of the total daily dose

Examples of these calculations can be seen in Table 13.2.

Once the total amount for the basal rate has been established, this should then be divided by 24 to give an hourly rate. Some insulin pumps have basal rates that can be programmed in increments of 0.05 or 0.025 units per hour;

**Table 13.2**   Calculation of initial basal rates

Pre-pump insulin dose = 9 units long-acting, 8 units rapid-acting insulin = 17 units
Reduce by 30% = 12 units as the total daily dose
Pre-school children: 4.2 units for the total basal rate (35%)
Pubescent children: 5.4 units for the total basal rate (45%)
Teenagers: 7.2 units for the total basal rate (60%)

others have 0.1 units per hour as the smallest increment. To avoid confusion, unless the pump is being used on a baby or small toddler, even if the pump has a basal rate that can be set in 0.025 unit increments it might be easier to use only one decimal place for the initial settings, saving the smaller increment differences for any fine-tuning required. More information on which basal rate increments are available for different pumps can be obtained from the pump manufacturers.

It might be possible to divide the basal rate exactly by 24 to give the same amount of insulin each hour, but this is unlikely, particularly when dealing with small insulin doses, so it might be necessary instead to give slightly more or less insulin for some hours of the day. Danne *et al.* (2005), looking at insulin doses used in children across 10 countries, found that preschool children often needed a lower basal rate in the early hours of the morning and that teenagers often needed a higher basal rate in those hours to combat the early-morning rise in blood glucose readings, although individuals' insulin needs will vary. It is important to remember that, whatever basal rate is chosen, this is just a starting point and is likely to need altering, so a close approximation to the dose required is likely to be sufficient at this stage.

Any alteration of the basal rate should be carried out on the basis of blood glucose results, with a clear agreement regarding the level of blood glucose to aim for. Chapter 11 provides guidance on how to agree what blood glucose levels to aim for in the first few days of starting to use a pump, and Chapter 10 provides information on how to alter basal rates in response to blood glucose readings. For babies and toddlers, the basal rates might need to be adjusted in increments of 0.05 units rather than 0.1 units per hour.

Using insulin pump therapy in children provides the opportunity to aim for tighter blood glucose control than might have been possible with injections, and NICE (2004) recommends that pre-prandial blood glucose levels of 4–8 mmol/l (millimoles per litre) should be aimed for in children and young people, although there might be variations for some individuals. If the child or parents have developed a fear of hypoglycaemia, which is common, the adjustment of the basal rate might need to be very gradual to achieve this.

On an ongoing basis, a child's insulin requirements are likely to change frequently, and the basal rates should be reviewed at every clinic visit, ideally every three months, to ensure they are optimally adjusted to help achieve the target blood glucose levels. Height and weight should be plotted on centile charts to ensure that the child is growing and developing normally, another indication of whether the insulin doses are close to requirements.

## Food boluses

As with adults, a standard food bolus rate of one unit of insulin to 10 grams of carbohydrate can usually be used as a starting point. However, if the pre-pump insulin doses are very small, a smaller amount of insulin to carbohydrate could be used. For example, a ratio of one unit to 20 grams of carbohydrate, or even one unit to 30 grams, might be used. Small babies might not require any boluses initially, as it might be possible to control their blood glucose level adequately by using the basal rate alone; in this age group, the regular use of continuous glucose monitoring sensors can help assess glycaemic control.

Because of hormonal changes, and also in those with a tendency towards high morning blood glucose levels as already discussed, some children will need different amounts of insulin to carbohydrate at different times of day. For example, they might need one unit to 8 grams of carbohydrate at breakfast time, one unit to 12 grams at lunchtime and one unit to 10 grams for their evening meal. Chapter Ten describes how blood glucose readings can be used to determine whether an alteration is needed to the insulin to carbohydrate ratio. If the ratio is worked out correctly, the blood glucose level two hours after giving the food bolus should be within 2 to 3 mmol/l of the pre-prandial level.

## Correction boluses

The amount of insulin a child will need to correct a high blood glucose level is likely to vary according to their age. As a general guide, for:

- children under 11 years of age, one unit will reduce their blood glucose by 5 mmol/l
- children aged 11 years or over, one unit will reduce their blood glucose by 2.5 mmol/l.

For babies or very small toddlers who require much smaller amounts of insulin, or those who are sensitive to small doses, the '100 rule' can be particularly

**Table 13.3** Using the 100 rule to calculate correction boluses

| |
|---|
| Total daily dose = 5 units |
| 100/5 = 20 |
| One unit of insulin will reduce the blood glucose by 20 mmol/l |
| Total daily dose = 20 units |
| 100/20 = 5 |
| One unit of insulin will reduce the blood glucose by 5 mmol/l |
| Total daily dose = 25 units |
| 100/25 = 4 |
| One unit of insulin will reduce the blood glucose by 4 mmol/l |

useful. Divide 100 by the total daily insulin dose, and this will provide the amount of millimoles that the blood glucose is likely to fall by when one unit of insulin is given. Examples can be seen in Table 13.3.

## CARBOHYDRATE ASSESSMENT

Assessing the amount of carbohydrate that is eaten is important at any age to be able to work out the appropriate insulin dose to give. Chapter Seven provides general information on how to approach this, including teaching carbohydrate assessment prior to starting to use a pump.

Information provided for children should be in a format that is easy to use, including pictures or photographs, to help them with recognising carbohydrate-containing foods and being able to assess quantities. Learning the amounts of carbohydrate in their most frequently eaten foods is the best starting point; anecdotally, children learn very quickly how much insulin they need to give for their favourite foods. They are likely to find it more difficult when faced with unfamiliar situations or foods, such as eating at a friend's house or going to a party, so planning ahead and liaising with friends' parents will help.

Children often snack between meals, and when using injection therapy they would not generally have given insulin at that point and so are likely to need reminders that they need to give a bolus for any snacks containing carbohydrate. They might also drink milk or orange juice on a regular basis and so, again, will need to give insulin for these types of drinks. Ketchup and other sauces are often consumed quite liberally, and these also need to be counted as part of the carbohydrate assessment. Clinic visits should include discussions about what tools children are using to assess their carbohydrate intake, and also identification of the level of success achieved by their efforts.

# DAY-TO-DAY PRACTICAL ISSUES

## Siting the infusion set

For older children, the infusion set can be sited in the abdomen or buttocks, as with adults, and in the same way the user will need to rotate their sites and ensure that they choose areas which will be comfortable in relation to the clothing they wish to wear. For babies, there could be very little subcutaneous tissue, and the thigh is likely to be the best site. For toddlers, once they are no longer wearing nappies, the buttock is the preferred site as it is out of sight and so is less likely to be interfered with by the child, and the tubing can also be safely tucked away.

Using the smallest needles and cannulae will mean that these areas can be safely used for most children, but for very small babies, who have minimal subcutaneous tissue, a hydrocolloid dressing can be applied to their skin first and then the smallest needle can be inserted through the dressing to ensure that it does not penetrate too deeply. Another option is to use a cannula designed for insertion at a 45-degree angle, inserting it at a 30-degree angle to penetrate less deeply, and also to not fully insert the cannula.

## Low insulin requirements

It has already been discussed that some children, particularly babies, are likely to need very small amounts of insulin. For some, even the lowest basal rates will be too high. In these cases, diluting the insulin is an option. Danne *et al.* (2005) suggest that dilution of U100 strength insulin might be necessary for the majority of preschool children in order to give accurate doses, but, in practice, insulin should not be diluted unless absolutely necessary, for a number of reasons. First, the insulin can only be used for a maximum of seven days before it expires, potentially creating additional work for the family. Second, the pump will provide information based on U100 insulin being used, so if different strengths of insulin are used the display on the pump will not match the amount of insulin being given. This means that additional calculations are required for every dose and there is greater potential for errors in dose calculation and adjustment.

If insulin has to be diluted, the safest way of ensuring the correct doses are given is to develop a chart with details of the insulin dose that is being delivered in relation to the reading on the pump. If the insulin is diluted to U50 strength, the pump would only be delivering half the dose indicated on the display, so a pump indicating delivery of 0.1 units of insulin would actually be delivering 0.05 units. If a dilution to U10 strength is used, the pump would deliver a tenth of the dose indicated on the display, so a reading of 0.1 units would actually deliver 0.01 units.

## Wearing the pump

Many pump manufacturers and other companies make a variety of clips and covers for insulin pumps, and children and young people are often keen to coordinate their pump cover with their clothes. Helping them gain access to a variety of covers for their pump can make this aspect of pump therapy fun. The pump manufacturers can provide some alternative pump covers, although these might need to be purchased at an additional cost. There are also a number of American websites where additional cases can be purchased (see the Appendix for more information). Alternatively, small purses, bags or a mobile phone cover might be used. For young children, sewing pockets into their clothes, for example their pyjamas or games kit, will keep the pump secure and avoid the need for a child to wear a pump cover. For toddlers, a small rucksack that can sit between their shoulder blades is the easiest method of carrying the pump, so that it reduces the chances of affecting the toddler's balance and also makes sure that the pump is out of the way and that the toddler won't interfere with it. Alternatively, attaching the case in the middle of a toddler's back by some other means is an option.

## Physical activity

Most activity undertaken by children is unplanned, such as running around the school playground, bike rides or an informal game of football after school. Different intensities of exercise can have profoundly different effects and are likely to require different management strategies. Developing an understanding of how different levels of activity affect a child's blood glucose levels, both at the time of the activity and for a number of hours afterwards, will help to determine how to manage their insulin and food.

For small children, eating additional snacks without giving an insulin bolus can be the simplest way of managing physical activity. Disconnecting the pump for short periods is also an option, to reduce the amount of insulin given. If the latter option is chosen, ideally the pump should be disconnected for no more than an hour. It should be kept in a clean and safe place to prevent damage or theft, or might be left with a teacher if at school. Also, the pump should be left in 'run' mode, as stopping the infusion will activate the alarm.

As children get older, a temporary basal rate can be used when physical activity is undertaken. Children can find this hard to remember when they are at school or away from their parents, although they might find it useful if they regularly need to make similar reductions in their insulin doses. If a reduced basal rate is required for part of the day, another option is to programme this into a completely separate basal rate and simply switch to that basal rate on the days when the reduction is needed, for example when there is a physical education or dance lesson. Again, this is not without difficulties: if the child does not undertake the activity for any reason, they are likely to have a higher blood glucose level than normal. Also, if changes are made to the basal rate for other reasons, such as balancing blood glucose levels overnight, the parents or child need to remember to alter both the normal basal rate and the one used for the physical education lesson.

As a general guide, snacks are an effective way of managing physical activity in most children if the activity is of short duration, for example 30 minutes or less. For longer periods, reducing the insulin dose by either disconnecting the pump or programming a reduced basal rate are more likely to be successful in keeping blood glucose levels balanced. Chapter 12 discusses the options for managing pump therapy in relation to physical activity more fully.

## Carrying supplies

Information on the day-to-day supplies required for a pump user is given in Chapter 12. For a small child, these supplies can be a lot to carry, and it would be useful to keep spare equipment in frequently attended places, such as at nursery, an after-school club or a best friend's house. Teenagers can be reluctant to carry large amounts of equipment around, and condensing their essential supplies as much as possible, plus thinking of innovative ways of carrying essential supplies, can help.

## Being away from home

Sleepovers, parties and school camps are usually attended by children without their parents, and many parents will commonly have anxieties about how their child will cope without them, particularly if they develop problems with their infusion site or are in situations where it is difficult for them to determine their precise insulin needs. Planning ahead is the key to success, and both parents and children might need help in working out how to deal with specific situations, particularly those they haven't previously encountered. Situations where a child will be more active, such as going away on a camp, are likely to require an overall reduction in insulin doses by around 10 to 20 per cent to avoid hypoglycaemia, although obviously individuals will vary. Depending on the age of the child, agreeing what can be coped with by them and what would necessitate a phone call home are all part of this planning process. The more prepared a child is – and the people who the child will be with – the better they will be able to manage the pump and enjoy the occasion along with their friends.

## Teenage years

Experimenting, rebelling against parental discipline and learning how to be independent are all part of normal teenage behaviour. Teenage years are also a period of growth and development, and calculating insulin doses to match daily requirements can be an arduous task. Significant insulin increases are often required in puberty, and basal rates might need to be set at one unit per hour or more. The regular review of basal rates at this time is important.

For girls, menstruation can affect their blood glucose levels, and in the early days periods are likely to be unpredictable. Many find they have higher blood glucose readings for one or two days before a period, and, if a pattern is established, this will help them to proactively adjust their insulin doses as required.

Keeping pace with changing insulin requirements through the teenage years can be a challenge, as the pump user can feel less inclined to put hard work into making their pump therapy work, preferring instead to be like their peers. Working with teenagers to agree simple sets of rules that can be adhered to, and agreeing how parents and health professionals can be involved and provide support, will help. Encouraging them to talk openly about any experimenting they are doing with their insulin doses and their diabetes, particularly when starting to drink alcohol, can help to maintain reasonable blood glucose levels and also keep the lines of communication open. More information about managing insulin doses in relation to alcohol can be found in Chapter Seven.

Telling a boyfriend or girlfriend about an insulin pump can be daunting. Teenage relationships are often transient, and it might not be necessary to have much discussion with a new partner about the pump, but it is important that the pump user does not try to be overly secretive about wearing the pump. This could lead to omitting boluses or even leaving the pump off when going on a date, resulting in hyperglycaemia and the potential risk of developing diabetic ketoacidosis. However, evidence suggests that ketoacidosis rates are lower in teenage pump users than those using injection therapy (Rodrigues *et al.*, 2005), so there is little likelihood of this happening. Exploring in consultations how teenagers will discuss their pump with prospective partners, including any concerns they have, will help them prepare for future relationships.

## INSULIN PUMPS AT SCHOOL

For school-age children, particularly those who are young, special consideration will need to be given to how their pump therapy is managed at school.
Providing the school with some general information about insulin pumps is a
useful starting point and giving a talk to the class the pump user is in can help
other children understand. Developing an individualised care plan in con-
junction with the school staff, and possibly the school nurse (although school
nurses are unlikely to have a major part to play, except possibly in special-
needs schools) is a key aspect of managing the pump during school time. The
Skills for Health Competency framework (Skills for Health, 2006), which outlines how to care for a child or young person with diabetes, provides general
information about what an individualised care plan should contain for any
child with diabetes and how the plan should be in line with the school's own
policies regarding aspects such as healthy eating, disability discrimination
and health and safety legislation. A summary of what an individualised care
plan should include is in Table 13.4.

One of the main issues to be considered is how to manage the lunchtime insulin bolus required. In some areas of the country, school staff are being taught
how to test blood glucose levels and give insulin by injection at lunchtimes,
to avoid the need for parents to visit the school on a daily basis, but this is still
relatively rare. If a child is able to press the buttons of their pump to give a
bolus of insulin, they might be able to give a fixed, agreed amount of insulin
with supervision, or, for young children, parents will still need to visit the
school each lunchtime to give a bolus dose. Taking packed lunches is the ideal
way for parents to calculate and control the amount of carbohydrate for their
child's midday meal. A child aged five or over might become familiar with
the carbohydrate content of some foods they regularly eat, for example the
type of crisps bought at home. They might even know how much insulin is

**Table 13.4**　Recommended contents of an individualised care plan for schoolchildren

---

Agreement about how frequently blood glucose levels should be tested, what levels are
acceptable and what action to take if the readings are higher or lower than the agreed
levels.

Arrangements for any supplies to be kept at school, and how they can be accessed.

How insulin doses will be calculated and what level of supervision the child needs.

How to manage sports or physical education lessons.

A communication plan regarding situations when the parents or carer should be alerted.

What to do in urgent situations, such as unresolved high blood glucose levels or infusion
site problems.

---

required when they eat the packet of crisps, but they will not be capable of more complex calculations that would be required if they ate less familiar foods.

If a more flexible system is required so that a child can choose which parts of their lunch they eat, parents could label foods according to how much insulin should be given for each item of food. This will enable the child to have snacks at break times and also decide for themselves how much lunch to eat, as other children may do, and give the correct insulin dose to match. For children who tend to eat varying amounts of their lunch, giving the insulin bolus after the meal is safest. If a child is not confident in giving a bolus, and parents are unable to visit the school each lunchtime, an alternative is to programme additional insulin into the basal rate at mealtimes, although this then means the child has no choice but to eat their lunch or snack.

It is rare for teaching staff to want to get involved in a major way, although they might be happy to supervise the amount of insulin being given in line with the written management plan. It is possible for schools to apply for additional funding to reflect the extra responsibility and supervision required for a child with diabetes.

A plan for physical activity is essential. As discussed in the 'Physical activity' section of this chapter, eating snacks for short periods or disconnecting the pump for sports or physical education lessons lasting longer than 30 minutes are effective management options.

Educating school staff and pupils is the key to success: the more they know, the more comfortable they will be with the pump, and they will be able to provide the child with support without being overanxious.

## ONGOING SUPPORT AND REVIEWS

Once a child has become accustomed to using an insulin pump, they should be reviewed as regularly as any other child with diabetes, a minimum of every three months. As already discussed, the review of basal rates and the proactive management of insulin doses are important, as their insulin requirements will be changing throughout their childhood and teenage years. Total basal rates and total daily doses of insulin should be checked, as this will help to identify whether the child is remembering to give boluses, whether they frequently need to give additional doses of insulin to lower their blood glucose levels and whether their day-to-day management should alter in any way. Centile charts are a good way of helping to assess whether a child is receiving enough insulin to be able to develop normally.

Asking a child to demonstrate how they handle their pump, and identifying how confidently they navigate the pump's menu systems, can show how comfortable they are with using the pump and also which functions are less familiar to them. As already discussed in this chapter, identifying what methods of carbohydrate assessment they are using, and discussing how well these methods are working, can help to increase their skill in this area.

If it is difficult to identify what is happening, or a child's glycaemic control is beginning to deteriorate, using a continuous glucose monitor sensor can help to identify trends and establish what changes need to be made. In babies and toddlers, continuous monitoring is likely to be needed relatively frequently to be able to establish what the optimum doses of insulin are.

It is important that the clinic review does not leave a child with a sense of failure or criticism. Providing praise where possible, celebrating successes and working with children and their parents to develop strategies to deal with situations that have been less successful are the most helpful approaches. It can also be a time for helping parents and children determine when parental control and input can be reduced and when a child might start to take on a more proactive role with the pump, keeping in mind that independence at too early a stage can be detrimental. It is perfectly acceptable for a child to take on a new responsibility one day and then ask their parent to be involved again the next, as it can indicate some uncertainty or possibly an inability to cope – discussing new responsibilities as 'experiments' can be helpful, as this doesn't instil a sense of failure if a child finds they don't cope as well as they expected. Sibling involvement is also important to enhance a sense of family unity and provide a better support system for the child using the pump.

It can be useful for children using insulin pumps to meet with their peers who also have diabetes – in some paediatric diabetes teams, groups are held specifically for pump users; in others, mixed groups of children using both pumps and injection therapy meet together. In either case, children are likely to be keen to swap experiences with others of a similar age, which can be the most effective way of developing new skills and different ways of managing situations. Whether this is part of a normal clinic structure or an addition to it, it is likely to maintain a child's interest and ongoing enthusiasm for managing their diabetes and their pump therapy proactively.

## CONCLUSION

This chapter has shown why insulin pump therapy is an important option that should be available to children and young people of any age. While many aspects of pump therapy are similar when dealing with children and adults, there are a number of significant differences. The key issues that affect children and insulin pumps have been discussed, particularly focusing on how much responsibility children should have at different ages and how the specialist diabetes team can work closely with a child and their parents, and also with the school, to help pump therapy be successful.

# REFERENCES

Bode BW, Steed RD, Davidson PC (1996) Reduction in severe hypoglycemia with long-term continuous subcutaneous insulin infusion in Type 1 diabetes. *Diabetes Care* **19**(4): 324–327.

Boland EA, Grey M, Oesterle A *et al.* (1999) Continuous subcutaneous insulin infusion: A new way to lower risk of severe hypoglycaemia, improve metabolic control and enhance coping in adolescents with type 1 diabetes. *Diabetes Care* **22**(11): 1779–1784.

British Nutrition Foundation (2004) Nutrition through life: School children, http://www.nutrition.org.uk/home.asp?siteId=43&sectionId=396&subSectionId=315&parentSection=299&which=1, accessed 22 May 2007.

Danne T, Battelino T, Kordonouri O *et al.* (2005) A cross-sectional international survey of continuous subcutaneous insulin infusion in 377 children and adolescents with type 1 diabetes mellitus from 10 countries. *Pediatric Diabetes* **6**(4): 193–198.

Department of Health (2001) *National Service Framework for Diabetes: Standards*, DH, London.

Greene S, Greene A (2005) Changing from the paediatric to the adult service: Guidance on the transition of care. *Practical Diabetes International* **22**(2): 41–45.

Hanas R, Adolfsson P (2006) Insulin pumps in pediatric routine care improve long-term metabolic control without increasing the risk of hypoglycemia. *Pediatric Diabetes* **7**(1): 25–31.

Heptulla RA, Allen HF, Gross TM, Reiter EO (2004) Continuous glucose monitoring in children with type 1 diabetes: Before and after insulin pump therapy. *Pediatric Diabetes* **5**(1): 10–15.

National Institute for Health and Clinical Excellence (2003) *Guidance on the use of continuous subcutaneous insulin infusion for diabetes*, NICE, London.

National Institute for Health and Clinical Excellence (2004) *Type 1 diabetes: diagnosis and management of type 1 diabetes in children, young people and adults*, NICE, London.

Rodrigues IAS, Reid HA, Ismail K, Amiel SA (2005) Indications and efficacy of continuous subcutaneous insulin infusion (CSII) therapy in Type 1 diabetes mellitus: A clinical audit in a specialist service. *Diabetic Medicine* **22**(7): 842–849.

Skills for Health (2006) Diab CYP13 Ensure the safety of a child/young person with diabetes in school, http://www.skillsforhealth.org.uk/tools/view_framework.php?id=110, accessed 13 June 2007.

# Chapter 14
# Insulin Pumps in Pregnancy

It is imperative to achieve tight glycaemic control in pregnancy to reduce the risk of maternal and fetal morbidity and mortality. Intensively managing diabetes during pregnancy is not a new concept and has been highlighted in many key and influential documents, including the *St Vincent Declaration* (Krans *et al.*, 1992) and the *Diabetes National Service Framework* (Department of Health, 2001). Despite this awareness, and the number of years that have passed since these major publications, the Confidential Enquiry into Maternal and Child Health (CEMACH) report into pregnancy care and outcomes in diabetes in England, Wales and Northern Ireland (Confidential Enquiry into Maternal and Child Health, 2007) has demonstrated that specialist services are failing to provide adequate pre-pregnancy counselling, and are also failing to achieve good glycaemic control before and during early pregnancy and during labour and delivery.

This chapter will first look at the advantages of using insulin pumps in pregnancy, including both the evidence base and experiences that are influencing practice in the United Kingdom. Following this, specific considerations relating directly to pregnancy will be covered, including initiating pump therapy, day-to-day practicalities and how to use pumps during labour. Post-delivery management and how to adjust insulin doses when breastfeeding will also be discussed.

## RATIONALE FOR PUMP USE DURING PREGNANCY

As discussed earlier in this book, insulin pumps can give people more flexibility and the opportunity to gain tighter glycaemic control, important considerations during pregnancy. The criteria for assessing suitability for using an insulin pump in pregnancy are the same as for non-pregnant women with diabetes, but there are also a number of additional benefits, which will be discussed in the remainder of this section.

## The need for tight glycaemic control

There is limited evidence around achieving tighter glycaemic control through the use of insulin pumps in pregnancy, although this could be due to the lack of large enough studies in this area. Studies suggest that the same level of glycaemic control can be achieved during pregnancy with multiple-dose insulin therapy rather than an insulin pump, using four or more injections per day, but these studies also suggest that if intensive therapy does not achieve the desired level of glycaemic control then an insulin pump is the treatment of choice (Burkart *et al.*, 1988). The advantages are that it has much less variation of absorption than conventional insulin regimens (Lauritzen *et al.*, 1983), that the slow infusion of insulin means there is very little subcutaneous depot of insulin, which reduces the risk of hypoglycaemia (Jornsay, 1998) and that the reduced variation between individual blood glucose readings (Wredling *et al.*, 1997) can help eliminate prolonged periods of hyperglycaemia.

## Reducing the risk of congenital malformations

There is ample evidence that poor glycaemic control in the pre-conception period, and in the early stages of pregnancy, is a major contributor to fetal congenital abnormalities (Confidential Enquiry into Maternal and Child Health, 2005). More recent evidence highlights that, despite this knowledge, two-thirds of women with diabetes have suboptimal glycaemic control before and during pregnancy (Confidential Enquiry into Maternal and Child Health, 2007). Tight glycaemic control is difficult to achieve at any time, and while pregnancy is often a time of high motivation to self-care the number of people who are not achieving glycaemic targets suggests that pump use is likely to be of benefit, although, as already discussed, evidence is limited in this area.

## Reducing severe hypoglycaemia

The evidence for insulin pump use reducing the incidence of severe hypoglycaemia has already been discussed in Chapter Two. Pregnancy carries a high risk of severe hypoglycaemia, which can be reduced through better glycaemic management. Even people who had sufficient glycaemic control previously might still benefit from using an insulin pump during pregnancy to be able to gain tighter glycaemic control with less hypoglycaemia. Being able to closely match the basal rate to insulin requirements can provide precise overnight control and so reduces the risk of night-time hypoglycaemia.

## Avoidance of ketoacidosis

While the incidence of ketoacidosis is low in pregnancy, it carries a high risk to the fetus, with up to 50 per cent fetal mortality (Jornsay, 1998). It is therefore important to be able to closely match insulin doses with requirements, which is easier to achieve when using an insulin pump than when using multiple-dose insulin therapy. As pregnancy progresses, when insulin resistance increases and large insulin doses are required, absorption using conventional insulin therapy becomes more erratic; by using a pump, the basal rate can be adjusted precisely to maintain tight glycaemic control.

## Management of morning sickness and delayed gastric emptying

Managing morning sickness and diabetes is problematic, as nausea and vomiting can make it difficult to eat in the mornings, and also cause problems when trying to treat hypoglycaemia. With insulin pump therapy, the basal rate can be adjusted, and boluses can be given in small increments to maintain good glycaemic control without hypoglycaemia. Also, pregnancy often causes delayed gastric emptying, which can be managed by using the prolonged bolus functions to match food absorption and also reduce post-prandial hyperglycaemia (Gabbe, 2000).

## WHEN TO START USING PUMP THERAPY

The use of insulin pumps in pregnancy varies across the United Kingdom. In centres where pumps are advocated for use in pregnancy, they are more likely to be considered at the pre-conception stage, if people with diabetes are able to access care at this point. The CEMACH report on diabetes and pregnancy (Confidential Enquiry into Maternal and Child Health, 2007) identifies that many people are poorly prepared for pregnancy, and most receive no pre-conception care, so it is not always possible to plan ahead this effectively. In areas where pumps are used less, they might only be used if adequate glycaemic control cannot be achieved using intensive insulin regimens.

## Pre-conception pump initiation

Ideally, if pumps are to be used during pregnancy, their use should be initiated prior to the pregnancy (Gabbe, 2000). If at all possible, this should be carried out six months prior to the pregnancy. This gives time to slowly improve glycaemic control, as rapid improvements are likely to accelerate any existing retinopathy. Also, anecdotally many pump users report that it takes about six months to gain full confidence with a pump and be able to work out what to do in all the different situations they encounter, as well as being more familiar with the pump functions that they don't necessarily use on a daily basis.

## Pump initiation during pregnancy

Experienced specialist teams in the United Kingdom report that they theoretically avoid initiating pump therapy in the first trimester, as they do not want to introduce a period of less good glycaemic control, which might increase the risk to the fetus of congenital malformations. However, if someone already has poor glycaemic control, they would be likely to initiate pump use during this period as glycaemic control is likely to improve, whereas if glycaemic control were reasonable, they would probably wait until around 12 weeks' gestation before using a pump. As health professionals become more experienced in pump management, confidence is likely to increase and initiating therapy early in pregnancy could become more common, ensuring strategies are in place to avoid ketoacidosis.

## SETTING AND ADJUSTING INSULIN DOSES

The usual way of calculating insulin starting doses for a pump is based on the total insulin dose prior to pump use, reducing this by around 30 per cent and then programming a proportion of that (around 50 per cent) as the basal rate, as described in Chapter 10. For someone who is pregnant, a smaller reduction in the total insulin dose might be considered, possibly around 15 to 20 per cent, to avoid hyperglycaemia and the risk of ketoacidosis and also to gain tight glycaemic control quickly during pregnancy. Around 60 per cent of the total should then be programmed as the basal rate, a slightly higher percentage than for those who are not pregnant.

It is important to consider that a rapid tightening of glycaemic control can worsen complications such as retinopathy (Diabetes Control and Complications Trial Research Group, 1993). Alongside this, the tightening of control is important to protect the fetus, so insulin doses should be adjusted more quickly than in someone who isn't pregnant. Fundoscopy prior to pump initiation and at regular intervals can help to identify problems early, and also prompt referral to more specialist ophthalmologic care should be available.

Regarding food and correction boluses, standard ratios can be used for pump initiation (as described in Chapter 10): one unit of insulin per 10 grams (or 1 CP) of carbohydrate and one unit of insulin to reduce the blood glucose level by 2.5 mmol/l (millimoles per litre). If the pump is being initiated later in pregnancy, these ratios can still be used but might quickly need revising on the basis of the blood glucose readings obtained.

As pregnancy progresses, insulin needs will increase incrementally, particularly towards the end of the second trimester and into the third. The doses required will vary from one person to another, but it is important to be proactive and regularly review both basal and bolus rates. Anecdotally, many women are reluctant to increase their insulin doses as quickly as their blood glucose readings suggest they should, so help and encouragement will be required to achieve this.

## Basal rate increases

Small changes in the basal rates are likely to be required initially, although this will accelerate, and in the third trimester incremental increases of 0.2 units per hour might be needed. Insulin resistance can often be seen more markedly early in the morning, because of the effect of placental hormones, and higher basal rates are likely to be needed at this time compared to the rest of the day.

## Food and correction bolus increases

Insulin to carbohydrate ratios are likely to change significantly, in line with basal rate requirements. Bolus requirements at breakfast might be twice as high as those required during the rest of the day by the end of pregnancy. It can also be helpful to use extended and mixed boluses to manage the delayed gastric emptying often experienced at this time. As with other dose adjustments, alterations to bolus calculations need to be tailored to the individual, based on their blood glucose levels.

Opinions vary regarding how correction boluses should be increased, as the level of blood glucose and also the time of day can influence the size of the correction bolus required. As a general guide, the '100 rule' can be used: divide 100 by the total daily insulin dose, and the resulting figure is the amount by which the blood glucose will be reduced by giving one unit of insulin. As an example, if the total daily insulin dose is 75 units, $100/75 = 1.5$, so one unit of insulin would be expected to reduce the blood glucose level by 1.5 mmol/l. In practice, the majority of people use less precise measures, but the 100 rule can be particularly useful in pregnancy as it takes into account the increasing insulin resistance and insulin doses. It can also be used as a reference point, to check whether the correction ratio correlates with this calculation, which will give some indication as to whether the doses being given are likely to be effective.

# PRACTICALITIES

Pump management in pregnancy needs to be very proactive, for the reasons already discussed. If insulin pump therapy is initiated in group education sessions, this method can still be used in pregnancy, but the amount and intensity of support following initiation will need to be greater. Weekly appointments with the specialist team, plus ideally a phone call during the week, and easy access if the pump user has queries should be provided. This will allow the early identification of any difficulties, as well as ensuring that insulin doses are increased at an early stage when blood glucose readings start to rise. As already discussed, many women who are pregnant can be reluctant to increase the dose quickly enough, and will need help and encouragement to feel confident in doing this.

## Management of infusion sites

The infusion set can still be sited in the abdomen, and many women prefer to continue with this, although as the pregnancy progresses the cannula or needle might need to be sited more laterally to be comfortable. Alternative sites such as the buttocks and thighs can be used, although help might be needed to insert the cannula or needle. Because the skin is stretched, angled cannulae rather than those inserted at 90 degrees can be safer as they are less likely to become dislodged.

The infusion set should be changed at least every 48 hours to ensure adequate absorption and so maintain tight glycaemic control. If blood glucose levels appear to be rising towards the end of the time the infusion set is being used, that suggests it needs changing more often. Also, the infusion set should be changed if two unexplained high blood glucose readings occur in succession, suggested by Gabbe (2000) as being above 11 mmol/l, to ensure adequate absorption.

If pump therapy is to be continued during labour, it is important that the partner or others who are present are taught how to change the infusion set. Trying this out early in the pregnancy will help them gain confidence to be able to manage it with competence during labour, and these skills will need to be revisited from time to time during the pregnancy.

## Blood glucose testing

Blood glucose testing should ideally be carried out at least eight times a day, to provide sufficient information to quickly identify any rising trends and adjust the insulin dose accordingly. Testing in the middle of the night should also be a regular part of management, particularly during the third trimester, to ensure that the night-time basal rate is keeping blood glucose levels under control. With such frequent testing, it is important not to overcorrect high blood glucose levels, as this is likely to precipitate hypoglycaemia. Correction boluses should be given no more frequently than one and a half hours apart, and ideally two hours.

## Ketone testing

Testing for ketones is important, using a meter to test for blood ketones rather than relying on urine testing. Testing for ketones is recommended when the blood glucose is around 10 mmol/l or higher, as ketones are likely to appear at a lower level in pregnancy. If ketones are present, a correction bolus should be given with a syringe or pen, and it is good practice to also change the infusion site and the infusion set at this point. However, ketones can also occur because the transfer of glucose across the placenta to the fetus can cause a rapid drop in the woman's blood glucose level, which can contribute to rapid fat metabolism and produce ketones as a result (Jornsay, 1998). This is most likely to happen during a period of fasting or when morning sickness occurs. If ketones appear when blood glucose levels are normal, this process should be suspected, and additional insulin is unlikely to be required, but frequent blood glucose testing should be carried out to ensure that insulin doses are closely matched to needs and that any increase in blood glucose levels can be quickly treated if it does occur.

## Carrying additional supplies

It is important to take adequate steps to ensure that blood glucose levels do not rise too high. If the pump is disconnected, this should be for short periods only, and for a maximum of one hour in every 24 hours. Also, additional supplies should be carried at all times, including insulin pens and needles, long-acting insulin and contact numbers for emergency care, as well as the equipment that is usually carried (as described in Chapter 12).

## Use of steroids during pregnancy

Steroid injections, usually two injections at 24-hour intervals, may be given antenatally if it is anticipated that the baby will be delivered at less than 36 weeks' gestation, as this will help the baby's lungs to mature. When the first injection is administered, the basal rate should be increased to 150 per cent, either by using the temporary basal rate or by programming a second basal rate and then switching to that when the dose of steroids is given. When the second injection of steroids is given, if the blood glucose level rises, the basal rate will need to be further increased, in 10 to 20 per cent increments, until blood glucose levels are under control.

Insulin to carbohydrate ratios and correction ratios will also be altered, and boluses around 50 per cent higher than usual are likely to be needed. Blood glucose levels will start to reduce 48 hours after the first injection, and the basal rate can gradually be reduced to its previous levels.

## Discontinuation of insulin pump therapy

If the pump user has to revert to injection therapy at any time during pregnancy, the formula described in Chapter 12 can still be used, but it might be difficult to calculate the insulin doses required, as insulin needs are constantly changing. The pump memory can be helpful for reviewing total daily basal and bolus doses over the preceding few days, to calculate the total daily doses of insulin. Ongoing written records of basal and bolus doses should also be encouraged throughout the pregnancy.

If a conversion chart for discontinuing pump therapy is used, this should be reviewed at least fortnightly to ensure it keeps pace with increasing insulin needs. Alternatively, a generic conversion chart containing insulin doses that match increasing needs could be developed and used throughout pregnancy. Access to a spare pump should also be considered in case of pump failure. This might be achieved by having a central place where a spare pump is kept, for example a hospital ward or a drop-in centre where access can be gained at any time.

## Preparation for labour

Early preparation for labour can be helpful. Any time after 30 weeks' gestation, a plan should be put in place and written in the medical notes of how labour should be managed, as detailed in the next section of this chapter. A second basal rate should be programmed into the pump for use after delivery of the baby. If the pump was initiated pre-pregnancy, the pump can be programmed with the basal rates that were used at that time. If not, the pre-pregnancy total daily insulin dose can be used as a guide, and around 50 per cent of that should be programmed as the basal rate. An alternative emergency plan should also be documented in the medical notes in case there is any reason why insulin pump therapy cannot be continued throughout labour.

It is also important at this stage to check that the partner, or whoever is likely to be present during labour, is familiar with programming the pump and changing the infusion set. Both the medical notes and the hand-held antenatal notes should contain the contact details for the insulin pump team in case their input is required.

## Pump supplies for during labour

Additional plans need to be made for using the pump to ensure adequate emergency supplies are brought to the hospital for use during labour. Table 14.1 provides information on what supplies should be available. Agreement should be gained that hypoglycaemia can be treated with glucose tablets or glucose gel, even if no food or drink are allowed otherwise, and this should be documented in the notes.

## LABOUR

As described earlier, pumps can safely be used in labour, providing the benefit of being able to alter the insulin dose very quickly in response to blood glucose readings, however prolonged labour is. Using pumps during labour instead of intravenous insulin regimens has been shown to provide better glycaemic control in this period, less fetal distress and also a lower incidence of hypoglycaemia in newborn babies (Feldberg *et al.*, 1988), so reducing the

**Table 14.1** Recommended additional supplies for during labour

- spare batteries for the pump
- spare insulin cartridge
- spare infusion sets
- blood ketone meter and testing strips
- glucose tablets or glucose gel

chances of the baby requiring treatment in a special care baby unit. Using pumps during labour also helps women feel more in control and less anxious about their diabetes management during labour, which provides flexibility and avoids having an intravenous infusion of dextrose and insulin. However, some women might choose to discontinue the pump during the early stages of labour – if this is the case, an intravenous infusion of insulin should be commenced.

## Siting of the needle or cannula

The needle or cannula should be sited out of the way during labour (avoiding the lower abdomen and the thighs as the tubing could get in the way during the birth) for example the upper arm or high on the lateral aspects of the abdomen will help ensure it does not cause problems, even if a Caesarian section is required. The infusion site should be changed every 24 hours if labour is prolonged.

## Pump management during labour

Self-management of the pump can be continued during labour, but in most cases the partner or other accompanying person is likely to play a large part in monitoring blood glucose levels and managing insulin doses and also might need to resite the needle or cannula, so they should be prepared to play this part as described in the previous section of this chapter. Hourly blood glucose readings, or using a continuous glucose monitoring system, mean that insulin doses can be finely tuned, and correction boluses of insulin should be given if blood glucose levels are above 7 mmol/l, to maintain tight glycaemic control.

Hospital policies, and the confidence or level of knowledge about insulin pumps, can influence whether the pump is continued during labour. Most hospital staff will be more familiar with intravenous insulin being used with a sliding scale and might raise concerns about a pump being self-managed once labour has commenced. Having a clear plan in the hospital notes and also the personal antenatal notes, and also liaising with the multidisciplinary team, including midwives, obstetricians and anaesthetists, prior to labour commencing will help. Education sessions can be held for staff working in obstetric units, but their lack of experience with insulin pumps can mean that they still lack confidence. The safest approach is to allow named individuals only to manage the pump during labour, for example the woman with diabetes, their partner, the diabetes team and possibly individuals within other disciplines if they have the confidence and experience to do this.

The pump can be discontinued at any time, either because of personal preference or if the obstetric team has concerns. The main reasons for removing pumps during labour would be:

- if women or their partners are finding it too much to cope with and can't concentrate on making the decisions they need to about managing the pump as well as dealing with the labour
- if blood glucose targets of 4–7 mmol/l are not being achieved
- if more than a trace of ketones is present in the blood.

If the pump is discontinued during labour, an intravenous infusion of insulin should be used.

## Reducing the insulin dose prior to the birth

Reducing the insulin dose is important during the later stages of labour, to avoid hypoglycaemia. The basal rate should be reduced to 80–90 per cent once active labour has commenced. When the second stage of labour begins, a further 10–20 per cent reduction should be programmed into the pump, using the temporary basal rate. Hourly blood glucose monitoring should be carried out throughout labour, and correction boluses should be given during labour if the blood glucose is above 7 mmol/l at any time. The pre-programmed second basal rate should be switched to when the baby is delivered.

## Caesarian section

If a Caesarian section is required, ideally epidural anaesthesia should be used, the pump should be kept on and can be managed by the pump user and her partner. If a general anaesthetic is needed, hospital policies vary regarding whether they will allow a pump to be used, which to some extent can depend on the experience and confidence of the anaesthetists and whether pumps are usually continued when other operations are carried out. Some hospitals allow the pump to be continued, using the basal rate, with frequent blood glucose checks and with the option of switching to an intravenous insulin regimen if the blood glucose is not well controlled. In practice, because the time under general anaesthetic is relatively short compared to many other operations, a blood glucose reading taken on arrival in theatre and another post-delivery is usually sufficient to identify whether good glycaemic control is being achieved. If the pump is to be kept on while under general anaesthesia, the insulin dose should be reduced to 90 per cent shortly before going to theatre, with a further reduction to 70–80 per cent just prior to going into theatre, and a further 10 per cent reduction might be required while in theatre. As with a vaginal delivery, the pump should be switched to the pre-programmed second basal rate when the baby is delivered. If the pump has been removed for the operation, it can be reconnected after recovery from the anaesthetic.

## POST DELIVERY

Most women are extremely keen to keep using an insulin pump, as it not only provides better glucose control but also allows them more flexibility in their lifestyles (Gabbe, 2000), and guidance from the Insulin Pumps Working Group (Department of Health, 2007) states that, once someone is initiated on an insulin pump, it is not good practice to take it away after delivery. For a small number, injections will be the preferred treatment, usually because they feel that intensively managing their diabetes as well as coping with a newborn baby is too much. In most centres, women are given the choice of continuing using a pump, although criteria might be set to measure whether their diabetes management remains optimal in order to justify continued pump use.

If the decision is made to discontinue the pump post delivery, the total daily dose of insulin before labour commenced should be the starting point; this should be reduced by 30 per cent (or 50 per cent if breastfeeding, as less insulin is needed), and then divided into four equal doses as a starting point for a basal bolus regimen, although most will continue to use insulin to carbohydrate ratios to decide how much insulin to have with their meals.

## BREASTFEEDING

Many women find breastfeeding much easier when using a pump, because of the increased flexibility and also because they are able to precisely alter their insulin doses to match their needs. These include having a lower basal insulin requirement, a need to increase the amount of carbohydrate eaten and avoidance of hypoglycaemia at feeding times. Blood glucose levels tend to be lower around the time of breastfeeding, despite women reporting a high calorie intake (Ferris *et al.*, 1988), but if blood glucose levels can be well controlled milk production and quality are enhanced, therefore increasing the chances of the mother being able to breastfeed (Abayomi *et al.*, 2005).

Overall insulin requirements will be much lower for breastfeeding women, so a basal rate lower than pre-pregnancy, or lower than 50 per cent of the pre-delivery dose, will be required. Around 30 per cent of the pre-delivery dose is a good starting point.

It is estimated that women lose around 40 to 50 grams of carbohydrate per day via breastfeeding (Department of Health, 1995) and so need to eat this amount of carbohydrate in addition to their usual dietary intake. However, the amount of insulin required for this will vary, as insulin requirements are lower at the actual time of breastfeeding. To avoid hypoglycaemia, women should test their blood glucose prior to feeding and correct any low blood glucose levels by eating carbohydrate without additional insulin. If their blood glucose level is within the desired range and they wish to snack, a reduced insulin to carbohydrate ratio should be used – possibly around 50 per cent of the amount of insulin to carbohydrate required at other times of the day. Most women are likely to need snacks around the time of breastfeeding to avoid hypoglycaemia but can be reluctant to eat extra food if they are trying to regain their pre-pregnancy weight; therefore, this advice might need to be reinforced on a regular basis.

## CONCLUSION

This chapter has identified and explored the many ways in which pump therapy can have a beneficial effect when used during pregnancy, and during the pre-conception period where possible. How to adjust insulin doses to closely match the varying needs for insulin during pregnancy and labour have been discussed, as well as specific issues that need to be addressed to ensure that tight glycaemic control is maintained at all times. Management of the pump during labour and also following delivery, particularly when breastfeeding, has been highlighted and specific issues addressed. In line with the general increase in pump use in the United Kingdom, given the benefits outlined here, the use of pump therapy in pregnancy is likely to increase as the confidence of health professionals grows in how to manage it.

## REFERENCES

Abayomi J, Morrison G, McFadden K *et al.* (2005) Can CSII assist women with type 1 diabetes in breastfeeding? *Journal of Diabetes Nursing* **9**(9): 346–351.
Burkart W, Hanker JP, Schneider HPG (1988) Complications and fetal outcome in diabetic pregnancy. *Gynecologic and Obstetric Investigation* **26**(2): 104–112.
Confidential Enquiry into Maternal and Child Health (2005) *Pregnancy in Women with Type 1 and 2 Diabetes*, CEMACH, London.
Confidential Enquiry into Maternal and Child Health (2007) *Diabetes in Pregnancy: Are We Providing the Best Care?*, CEMACH, London.

Department of Health (1995) *Breastfeeding: Good Practice Guidance to the NHS*, DH, London.

Department of Health (2001) *National Service Framework for Diabetes: Standards*, DH, London.

Department of Health (2007) *Insulin Pump Services*, DH, London.

Diabetes Control and Complications Trial Research Group (1993) The effect of intensive treatment of diabetes on the development and progression of long-term complications in insulin-dependent diabetes mellitus. *New England Journal of Medicine* **329**(14): 977–986.

Feldberg D, Dicker D, Samuel N *et al.* (1988) Intrapartum management of insulin-dependent diabetes mellitus (IDDM) Gestants: A comparative study of constant intravenous insulin infusion and continuous subcutaneous insulin infusion pump (CSIIP). *Acta Obstetricia et Gynecologica Scandinavica* **67**(4): 333–338.

Ferris AM, Dalidowitz CK, Ingardia CM *et al.* (1988) Lactation outcome in insulin-dependent diabetic women. *Journal of the American Dietetic Association* **88**(3): 317–333.

Gabbe SG (2000) New concepts and applications in the use of the insulin pump during pregnancy. *Journal of Maternal-Fetal Medicine* **9**(1): 42–45.

Jornsay DL (1998) Continuous subcutaneous insulin infusion (CSII) therapy during pregnancy. *Diabetes Spectrum* **11**(suppl. 1): 26–32.

Krans HMJ, Porta M, Keen H (1992) *Diabetes Care and Research in Europe: The St Vincent Declaration Action Programme*, World Health Organisation, Regional Office for Europe, Copenhagen.

Lauritzen T, Pramming S, Deckert T, Binder C (1983) Pharmacokinetics of continuous subcutaneous insulin infusion. *Diabetologia* **24**(5): 326–329.

Wredling R, Hannerz L, Johannson U-B (1997) Variability of blood glucose levels in patients treated with continuous subcutaneous insulin infusion: A pilot study. *Practical Diabetes International* **14**(1): 5–8.

# Chapter 15
# Situations Requiring Complex Management

This chapter discusses a number of situations that require careful management when using insulin pump therapy. These include the action required to deal with illness, the prevention and treatment of ketoacidosis and management on admission to hospital, including when general anaesthesia is required. Specific conditions that complicate diabetes management but where pump use can be helpful are then looked at, which are: renal failure (including management of dialysis), gastroparesis and cystic fibrosis. The information presented here is for general guidance only and will need to be adapted when managing different conditions, as professional experience is relatively limited in these areas and research is required to identify what might in the future be considered good practice.

## ILLNESS

It is particularly important to proactively manage insulin pump therapy during illness, as the absence of longer-acting insulin can mean that blood glucose levels will potentially rise very quickly. The most important aspect is to ensure that enough insulin is being infused to prevent ketoacidosis, discussed later in this chapter. It is likely that illness-related hyperglycaemia will need a number of strategies to manage it effectively. Table 15.1 provides a summary of the potential action that will be required, and the following sections discuss the management of illness in more detail.

### Correction boluses

Blood glucose levels should be checked at the first sign of illness, for example if a cough, cold or raised body temperature develops, and a correction dose

**Table 15.1**   Potential action to take during illness

- Give correction boluses at two-hourly intervals in response to hyperglycaemia
- Temporarily increase the basal rate
- Test for ketones and take action if they are present
- Ensure infusion site is not infected or inflamed
- Change infusion site if blood glucose remains high
- Consider giving correction boluses by syringe or insulin pen
- Seek medical help promptly if treatment appears ineffective

of insulin should be given if the blood glucose is above the target range. Blood glucose levels should be tested at two-hourly intervals, with additional correction doses given if the blood glucose continues to be above the target range. Chapter 10 provides more information about calculating correction boluses.

If a pump user has a level of hyperglycaemia that is causing them significant concern, they might wish to test their blood glucose more frequently than every two hours, to establish whether the correction dose is working. While this can provide useful information, it also has drawbacks, as the pump user might be tempted to give additional correction boluses close together. They should be encouraged to give correction boluses at least one and a half hours apart, and ideally two hours, as boluses given too frequently are likely to have a cumulative effect that then carries the risk of inducing hypoglycaemia.

## Basal rate adjustment

If more than a single correction dose is needed when unwell, temporarily increasing the basal rate should also be considered. This is because correction doses are only providing additional insulin to treat the raised blood glucose, but illness or a raised temperature is likely to cause insulin requirements to be raised for more than a 24-hour period. An increase in the basal rate will help to prevent a recurrence of the hyperglycaemia, as well as potentially reducing the number of correction doses that are required. As at any other time, it is important to take account of any carbohydrate consumed in the two hours prior to the blood glucose being measured, as any food boluses might not have had time to take full effect, which could mean there is some residual (and misleading) hyperglycaemia that does not require a correction bolus.

As a starting point, if the temporary basal rate feature is used, it should be increased to 130 per cent, thereby giving 30 per cent more insulin than usual, as well as giving correction doses. Two-hourly blood glucose measurements are required to assess the effect of this, and, if the blood glucose is at a similar level or higher after two hours, the rate should be further increased to 160 per cent, and additional increases in 30 per cent increments should be considered if hyperglycaemia occurs. If more than double the usual basal rate needs to be infused, this will be beyond the scope of the temporary basal rate settings, and the pump user will need to set a new basal rate to ensure enough insulin is delivered to be effective. Using an alternative basal rate is recommended for this, as the pump user then still has their pre-illness basal rate programme available and can revert back to it when required.

If the illness is prolonged, the higher basal rate might be needed for a number of days, and more frequent site changes might be required as a result of the higher doses of insulin being infused. Medical help should be sought if the additional insulin does not appear to be controlling blood glucose levels adequately enough.

Anecdotally, pump users are often reluctant to increase their basal rate in large enough quantities to be effective and often view increases to 150 per cent or more as being very high. In reality, the basal rate for most pump users is often set at less than one unit per hour, so even large percentage increases only provide small additional amounts of insulin. Hyperglycaemia caused by illness might need double, treble or quadruple the usual amounts of insulin to be effectively managed, and raising awareness of this fact in initial pump education can help pump users feel more comfortable about making significant basal rate increases when unwell.

## Ketone testing and management

As well as increasing basal rates and giving correction boluses, ketone testing should also be carried out when treating prolonged illness-related hyperglycaemia. Ketone testing should be carried out if the blood glucose level is still high two hours after the first correction dose is given, and, if ketones are present, higher levels of correction doses will be needed. See the 'Ketoacidosis' section later in this chapter for information on how to treat hyperglycaemia when ketones are present.

## Infusion site management

If ketones are present at any point, or if correction boluses and the increased basal rate do not appear to be taking effect, the pump user needs to ensure that insulin is being infused and absorbed properly. Checking the infusion site for any sign of redness or inflammation at an early stage is recommended, but even if this looks normal the cannula or needle might be damaged or blocked, so resiting is recommended. Also, giving correction doses with a syringe or pen is an alternative, to ensure the insulin is being delivered, until the blood glucose level has returned to close to the target range.

## Nausea and vomiting

If nausea and vomiting occur due to the person being unwell rather than because ketones are present, insulin should still be infused using the pump but care should be taken to avoid hypoglycaemia where possible, as the pump user might find this difficult to treat if they are feeling very nauseous. If blood glucose levels start to fall, a temporary basal rate decrease should be used. Frequent oral fluids should be encouraged, as dehydration can easily occur if the pump user is vomiting and also has hyperglycaemia. If the pump user is unable to eat or drink for more than 24 hours, they should either call the diabetes team or access medical advice to identify whether they need hospitalisation.

## Recovery from illness

Once the person starts to recover from their illness, blood glucose levels will start to fall. Once readings of around 6 mmol/l (millimoles per litre) are being achieved, the temporary basal rate should be reduced gradually, in 30 per cent increments, to avoid hypoglycaemia. Two-hourly blood glucose testing is still recommended at this stage, and, if the blood glucose starts to fall below 6 mmol/l, further reductions in the temporary basal rate will be required, until the pump user reaches their pre-illness basal rate.

## KETOACIDOSIS

It has already been stated, in Chapter One, that ketoacidosis is no more common in pump users than those using injection therapy, but it is still a risk. Ketones associated with high blood glucose levels are most likely to appear in the following situations:

- when blood glucose testing is reduced and a rise in blood glucose levels goes undetected
- when someone is testing their blood but not giving adequate correction boluses
- when someone is unwell for other reasons and blood glucose levels are inadequately managed
- when someone is taking less insulin than they need (e.g. by missing bolus doses or disconnecting the pump for too long).

The management of hyperglycaemia is discussed in Chapter 11, including doubling correction doses if ketones are present, and the basal rate should be increased as described earlier in the 'Illness' section of this chapter. If the blood glucose remains high two hours after a correction dose and ketones are still present, the pump user should give the next correction dose with a syringe or insulin pen, and again the amount required will be higher than the usual correction ratio. Doubling the correction dose might be enough, but very high blood glucose readings, for example above 20 mmol/l, are likely to need in excess of 10 units of insulin as a correction dose.

Fluid intake is crucial, and at least 500 ml (millilitres) of water or other sugar-free liquids should be drunk every hour. A new cannula should be inserted in a site away from the previous one, the pump settings should be checked and the tubing of the infusion set should be checked to ensure that it is infusing insulin without air bubbles. If there is no improvement in either blood glucose levels or in the reduction of ketones, medical help should be sought as an emergency.

## HOSPITAL ADMISSIONS

Hospital admissions often pose difficulties with diabetes, as there can be tension between the hospital staff's responsibility for the treatment they are administering and the need for someone with diabetes to self-manage their condition as far as possible. Pump therapy can successfully be continued in hospital, as long as the pump user is well enough to continue managing it. If the pump user is too unwell to manage their pump, injection therapy or intravenous insulin will need to be used, as most hospital medical and nursing staff will have little or no experience of insulin pump therapy. Once the person with diabetes feels better, pump therapy can be recommenced. Taking a proactive approach to using pumps in hospital will help this type of treatment be more readily accepted by hospital staff.

### Education and awareness of nursing and medical staff

Part of the specialist diabetes team's responsibilities include raising awareness across hospital and community health settings about pumps, but it is unrealistic to try and educate all health professionals to a standard where they will have an in-depth understanding of pump therapy or be able to manage it. If pumps are being used within a district, hospital policies and information sheets can be produced for wards and departments, to help health professionals understand the basic principles of pump therapy and the importance of the pump user managing it themselves.

For a planned admission, talking to the nursing and medical staff before-hand about continuing the pump will help overcome some of their potential lack of knowledge; this discussion might involve both the pump user and the specialist insulin pump team. Taking the pump instruction manual into hospital can be helpful, together with a conversion chart (based on insulin requirements at the time) in case it is necessary to revert to injection therapy for a short period of time.

For an emergency admission, it is less easy to plan ahead, but information about insulin pumps kept in departments such as accident and emergency can be helpful. Information about when to intervene can be included, for example if the pump user loses consciousness or any other situation develops where the pump has to be discontinued for a period of time. It is important that hospital staff are aware that any interruption of the insulin supply from a pump can result in major hyperglycaemia within a few hours and so, if the pump is removed, insulin should be replaced immediately with an alternative method, such as an intravenous infusion.

The pump needs to be removed for some investigations, for example X-rays, MRI scans and CT scans, although it can still be worn during ultrasound scans. Again, information about this can be kept in the relevant departments and also be given to pump users who need to undergo this type of investigation.

## General anaesthesia

For operations or procedures of short duration that require general anaes-thesia, there is no reason why an insulin pump should not be continued, as the basal rate will maintain glycaemic stability even if the pump user is not eating. Blood glucose readings should be checked in the operating theatre immediately prior to the operation and again at the end. If the procedure is more complicated, or if an operation is likely to take a number of hours, it is more prudent to use an intravenous infusion, as this can be managed by anaesthetic staff during the time the person is under general anaesthesia. For some operations, it could be a few days before the pump user is able to eat again, although they can revert back to pump use at whatever time they feel well enough to manage it, which might be before they start to eat.

## Conversion from intravenous insulin back to insulin pump use

If someone's diabetes has been treated with intravenous insulin during their hospital stay, at some point they will need to revert back to using their insulin pump again. Because intravenous insulin has a very short action, the subcutaneous insulin infusion via the pump should be initiated 30 minutes before the intravenous infusion is discontinued, to maintain adequate control of blood glucose levels.

## RENAL FAILURE

End-stage renal failure requires careful management to match changing insulin requirements. If insulin pump therapy is being initiated when the person with diabetes is already in end-stage renal failure, basal rates should be set very low initially, as the long-acting insulin from multiple-dose insulin therapy might continue working for up to a week.

If someone is already using a pump and then goes into end-stage renal failure, they will experience a major drop in insulin requirements and will need to make substantial changes to insulin doses, both basal and boluses. A temporary basal rate reduction can be used initially to assess how much reduction is required, but basal rates will need to be reset to the lower amounts required. It can be difficult for pump users to believe that such large decreases in their insulin doses are necessary, and careful discussion is likely to be needed, otherwise they will be at an increased risk of experiencing hypoglycaemia.

The management of any type of dialysis can be problematic. The first step is to ensure that the usual basal rate is titrated against blood glucose readings to gain glycaemic stability without hypoglycaemia. When undergoing dialysis, the pump user's usual insulin to carbohydrate ratio, and correction ratio, should continue to be used. It is also important to ensure that the pump user receives consistent messages, particularly about dietary management, and close liaison is likely to be required between diabetes and renal specialist dietitians to achieve this. The following sections outline the specific management required for different types of dialysis.

## Haemodialysis

Haemodialysis carries with it the risk of fluid overload, which can affect basal rate requirements. On the days when the pump user is undergoing dialysis, they should set their temporary basal rate at 50 per cent an hour before the dialysis commences to avoid hypoglycaemia. As soon as the dialysis is complete, the basal rate can be returned to the usual infusion rate.

## Peritoneal dialysis

Peritoneal dialysis is complex to manage, as the strength of the dialysing fluid will change at times depending on the pump user's needs, and also the dialysing cycle might vary. The basal rate requirements will be higher when dialysis is taking place, and over time it will be possible to programme in regular variations to the basal rates to match the times when dialysis is being performed. Overnight dialysis is easier to manage, as the timings of the dialysis session are likely to be more regular.

When higher- or lower-strength bags of dialysing fluid are used, insulin requirements will alter. If a higher strength than usual is used, insulin will need to be increased, ideally using the temporary basal rate, but it is also possible to manage this by giving correction boluses in response to hyperglycaemia. If a lower-strength fluid is used, a temporary basal rate decrease will be needed to prevent hypoglycaemia. Close blood glucose monitoring should be continued as ongoing adjustments to insulin doses are likely to be necessary. It is also important to choose an infusion site for the pump that is well away from the dialysis site.

## GASTROPARESIS

The main difficulty in managing gastroparesis is matching the delayed or erratic absorption of food, which is often completely unpredictable from one day to the next, with bolus insulin doses. Using an insulin pump can be helpful, as doses can be adjusted in small amounts, and also boluses can be tailored to potentially more closely match food absorption.

The first step is to try and ensure that the basal rate is set correctly, so that when no food is eaten the blood glucose levels stay within or close to the target range. Extended boluses over 30 minutes to two hours should be used for all carbohydrate-containing foods, even if the amount of carbohydrate is very small. This gives the pump user the opportunity to cancel the bolus in case of a lack of absorption of the food. It can be helpful for the specialist diabetes dietitian to work closely with the pump user in relation to food choices, to reduce the types of foods that might further delay gastric emptying because of their prolonged absorption time.

If glycaemic control improves, this can improve gastric emptying, which might mean that insulin is required more quickly with food boluses. If this appears to be the case, a small proportion – probably no more than 20 per cent – of the total bolus can be given as a standard bolus, with the remainder programmed as an extended bolus. As with other situations, blood glucose testing and an analysis of the results will help the pump user determine the most successful method of insulin administration.

## CYSTIC FIBROSIS

Treatment for cystic fibrosis often includes long-term treatment with oral steroids, and insulin requirements are likely to be significantly higher than for other people. In addition, illness, or treatment with intravenous antibiotics, can increase insulin requirements by up to four times. The temporary basal rate can be used initially when unwell, but as insulin requirements increase the basal rate is likely to need to be reprogrammed to be able to deliver enough insulin to meet requirements. Basal rates of more than two units per hour are likely to be needed as a routine, and in some cases they can be higher than 10 units per hour. Not all pumps can be programmed to accommodate such a high basal rate, and, if this is the case, additional insulin doses will need to be given regularly each hour.

When someone with cystic fibrosis is unwell, a higher number of correction boluses are likely to be needed to maintain blood glucose levels close to their target range, as well as increasing the basal rates. Correction ratios and insulin to carbohydrate ratios might be affected when steroids are being used, so blood glucose readings should be assessed to identify the optimum bolus ratios to use. Over time, patterns might emerge that will provide information on which to base insulin doses in different situations.

## CONCLUSION

This chapter has identified a number of situations where insulin pumps need to be managed differently from usual. There will be many other situations that can affect insulin requirements or absorption, and pump users should be encouraged to follow the general principles of pump management, to test their blood glucose levels frequently and respond to any changes by increasing and decreasing their insulin doses. If someone with diabetes has experience of altering their multiple-dose insulin therapy doses in relation to a specific situation, this knowledge can be adapted and used as a starting point for decisions about pump management.

Appendix
# Additional Sources of Information

The following are a selection of websites available that might be helpful for both health professionals and pump users.

## NICE guidance on the use of insulin pump therapy (continuous subcutaneous insulin infusion)
www.guidance.nice.org.uk/TA57/guidance/pdf/english

This outlines a summary of available evidence and the recommendations of what criteria should be used when assessing an individual's suitability to use insulin pump therapy.

## Insulin Pump Services: Report of the Insulin Pumps Working Group, 2007
www.dh.gov.uk/en/publicationsandstatistics/publications/
publicationspolicyandguidance/DH_072777

The working group was set up to address variation in access to insulin pump therapy across the country. The report outlines the group's conclusions and gives examples of best practice in improving access to pump therapy.

## Diabetes UK position statement on insulin pump therapy
www.diabetes.org.uk/about_us/our_views/position_statements/insulin_
pump_therapy

This provides information on the cost-effectiveness of insulin pump therapy and how NICE guidance on this topic might be implemented.

## PUMP: Pump Management for Professionals
www.insulin-pump.info

This site is run by health professionals involved in pump therapy, to provide a multidisciplinary forum for education and support and to promote more widespread use of insulin pumps in the United Kingdom. It provides general information about insulin pump therapy, plus guidance for management in specific clinical situations. PUMP also runs national conferences and study days for health professionals and can provide information on health professional courses available.

## INPUT
www.input.me.uk

INPUT is an independent organisation run by pump users and their families and was set up to raise awareness of insulin pump therapy and to support more widespread use of insulin pumps in the United Kingdom. The site provides information on insulin pumps, how to obtain them, how to approach funding issues and is also involved in national initiatives to develop policy that supports the appropriate use of insulin pumps. Roadshows and other meetings are also held at different places in the United Kingdom, and INPUT members will present to local meetings of people with diabetes and also to NHS organisations.

## Insulin Pumpers UK
www.insulin-pumpers.org.uk

Insulin Pumpers UK is an Internet-based group, run by volunteers, to promote the knowledge and use of insulin pumps in diabetes. It provides information on insulin pumps and their use and also has email discussion groups, both UK and international, for insulin pump users to ask questions and share information.

## Bournemouth Diabetes Learning Programme
www.bdec-e-learning.com

This is an interactive website produced by the Bournemouth diabetes team to help people with diabetes learn the principles of carbohydrate assessment and insulin adjustment.

## Children with Diabetes
www.childrenwithdiabetes.com

This is a comprehensive American website providing information about the use of insulin pumps in children.

www.childrenwithdiabetes.co.uk

This is a UK website providing information about the use of insulin pumps in children.

## Pump accessories websites

www.angelbearpumpwear.com
www.pumppack.com
www.pumpwearinc.com
www.insulinpumppacksforyou.com

These American websites offer various holders for insulin pumps, including pouches, belts, T-shirts with pouches and backpacks, for small children.

# Index